Weight Loss
Confidential

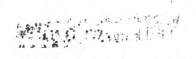

Weight Loss
Confidential

How Teens
Lose Weight and Keep It Off
—and What They Wish
Parents Knew

Anne M. Fletcher, M.S., R.D.

Foreword by Holly R. Wyatt, M.D.

HOUGHTON MIFFLIN COMPANY

BOSTON   NEW YORK

Copyright © 2006 by Anne M. Fletcher
Foreword copyright © 2006 by Holly R. Wyatt

Visit our Web site: www.houghtonmifflinbooks.com.

Library of Congress Cataloging-in-Publication Data

Fletcher, Anne M.
  Weight loss confidential: how teens lose weight and keep
it off— and what they wish parents knew / Anne M. Fletcher.
    p. cm.
  Includes index.
  ISBN-13: 978-0-618-43366-7
  ISBN-10: 0-618-43366-X
  1. Weight loss.   2. Weight loss— Case studies.
  3. Teenagers— Nutrition.   4. Reducing diets. I. Title.
  RM222.2.F537 2006
  613.2'5—dc22   2006016832

All trademarks are the property of their respective owners.

Book design by Anne Chalmers

Printed in the United States of America

MP 10 9 8 7 6 5 4 3 2

For WES,
whose journey inspired this book

For my other two teens, TY AND JULIA,
whose humor and spirit enrich my life

And for my mother-in-law, RUTH,
who's a teenager at heart

Acknowledgments

Writing a book like this is like making a big patchwork quilt: the efforts of countless other people make it all come together. Only the author can fully appreciate their benevolence.

First and foremost, my deep appreciation goes to the many teens and young adults—as well as their parents—who, in their willingness to help others, took the time to share their personal stories, complete a long questionnaire, and respond to my many e-mails and letters. In particular, the profiled teens and some of their parents devoted hours to telling me about their triumphs and tribulations. Special thanks go to my oldest son, Wes, who endured my best attempts at parenting—in and out of the kitchen—and whose experiences inspired this book. He is an amazing "kid" who can do just about anything he puts his mind to and was a good sport about sharing personal information and experiences throughout the book.

Next, my appreciation is extended to the scores of friends, teachers, counselors, relatives, high school principals, professors, YMCAs, colleagues, Web sites, and other organizations — too many to name — who helped me recruit young people for *Weight Loss Confidential.* I am indebted to the many weight programs, listed in "Weight Programs Used by the Teens," that went out of their way to help me find young people who would participate in the project. Thanks, too, to members of the American Dietetic Association's weight management and pediatric practice groups, which helped me recruit teens, as did Lee Dean at the *Minneapolis Star Tribune;* Rhoda Fukushima at the *St. Paul Pioneer Press; National Native News;* Natural Ovens Bakery; *New Moon* magazine; and the makers of Revival Soy.

The list of child and adolescent weight and obesity experts who responded to my many queries and reviewed sections of the book seems endless. I never cease to be amazed at how lucky I am to know experts willing to provide feedback for my books in progress. Special thanks go to Kerri Boutelle, Ph.D., an expert on adolescent weight issues and eating disorders at the University of Minnesota, who acted as a consultant for *Weight Loss Confidential* and became a supportive friend in the process. Stanford University's pediatric weight expert Thomas Robinson, M.D., was incredibly helpful by responding to countless e-mail questions, even when he was on vacation. Other frequent and appreciated respondents to my queries include James Anderson, M.D., of the University of Kentucky; William Dietz, M.D., Ph.D., director of the Centers for Disease Control and Prevention's Division of Nutrition and Physical Activity; Julie Germann, Ph.D., of La Rabida Children's Hospital in Chicago; Thomas Inge, M.D., Ph.D., of Cincinnati Children's Hospital Medical Center; Susan Johnson, Ph.D., of the University of Colorado Health Sciences Center; Thomas McKenzie, Ph.D., of San Diego State University; Dianne Neumark-Sztainer, Ph.D., R.D., of the University of Minnesota; Nancy Sherwood, Ph.D., of the HealthPartners Research Foundation in Minneapolis; and Jamie Stang, Ph.D., R.D., of the University of Minnesota.

Other experts who provided time and counsel include Arne Astrup, M.D., of Denmark's Royal Veterinary and Agricultural University; Sarah Barlow, M.D., of the St. Louis University School of Medicine; Susan Barr, Ph.D., R.D., of the University of British Columbia; Leann Birch, Ph.D., of Penn State University; Canice Crerand, Ph.D., of the University of Pennsylvania; John Foreyt, Ph.D., of the Baylor College of Medicine; Gary Foster, Ph.D., of Temple University; Daniel Kirschenbaum, Ph.D., of Northwestern University; Robert McMurray, Ph.D., of the University of North Carolina at Chapel Hill; Suzanne Phelan, Ph.D., and James Hill, Ph.D., researchers with the National Weight Control Registry; Barbara Rolls, Ph.D., of Penn State University; Dale Schoeller,

Ph.D., of the University of Wisconsin–Madison; and Eric Stice, Ph.D., of the University of Texas.

As with my previous books, I am indebted to my research assistant, Mary Stadick, and to Kristin Woizeschke, who keeps me stocked with journal articles. Several of my nutrition colleagues deserve special thanks for helping to develop the questionnaire that was sent to the teens: Ann Litt, M.S., R.D.; Helen Seagle, M.S., R.D.; and Lisa Talamini, R.D. Other questionnaire reviewers include high school counselor Sherryl Wolff, teacher Jane Schostag, and Lindsay Schostag. My friend and local high school principal John Barnett helped with the process, too. Behind the scenes, Lewis Robbins and Emily Neller, M.S., graciously provided editorial and research assistance.

My personal confidants and supporters throughout the three years that it took to write this book include Christine Kile, Roxie Meyer, Patty Christiansen, and Larry Lindner. Larry is always there and keeps reminding me that my readers will hear me better if I stop being "a scientist in a writer's body."

After doing five books with Rux Martin, I realize more than ever what a truly gifted editor she is. Rux appreciates my need to base my books on sound research findings, then helps me get out of my "scientist's body" to distill what's important and connect with my readers. It's hard to know how to thank my agent, Chris Tomasino, whose encouragement and willingness to do far more than the usual agent stuff goes beyond the call of duty. And even though he's no longer obligated, Barry Estabrook still provides wonderful editorial feedback, for which I am grateful.

Last but not least, I cannot express how much I appreciate my family — my husband, Steve, my three children, my mother and father, my mother-in-law, and my sisters — for putting up with my endless chatter and late nights working on this book. When they read the inspirational stories of the *Weight Loss Confidential* teens, they will know that it was all incredibly worthwhile.

Author's Note

Before starting any weight loss plan, diet, or exercise regimen, children and teens should seek the permission and supervision of their physicians, who may want to run medical tests to make sure a weight problem is not caused by a medical condition. They should also consult a physician before following the advice or guidelines in *Weight Loss Confidential*. This is particularly important for anyone with a medical condition such as diabetes or high blood pressure. A registered dietitian's counsel is advised as well. Overweight children and teens who are trying to reach a healthier weight should be monitored regularly by a physician to make sure they are healthy and growing properly. If a child or teen has or appears to have an eating disorder or is at risk for developing one, a physician and a licensed mental health professional should be consulted and can help determine whether the advice in this book is appropriate for the individual. This advice is also important if a child or teen is experiencing psychological distress, such as depression.

All the teens in *Weight Loss Confidential* have given their permission to share information about their weight histories. For those under the age of eighteen, their parents have given permission as well. Most of the names have been changed to protect the teens' privacy. Sometimes the teens' and their parents' remarks were edited slightly for clarity. Some of the facts in this book may have changed since the information was gathered.

Contents

Foreword

Not a single week passes that I don't read a major media story highlighting the epidemic of obesity our nation is facing and the serious repercussions this will have on our society's health. Most of us now realize that we're a fat society and getting fatter. Even more alarming is that the epidemic has not spared anyone — not even our children. The latest results from the National Health and Nutrition Examination Survey, the most accurate monitoring system for weight problems in the U.S. population, estimates that one third of children and adolescents ages two to nineteen are now overweight or at risk for being overweight. Public health professionals have worked hard to raise awareness of the issue and help us understand that the epidemic is real and has massive implications for our families and our children.

Okay, we're getting the message. Now what do we do about it? The fire alarm has been pulled, but where is the water? It's bad enough to frighten us with a problem and not give a solution. It's even worse to provide us with the statistics showing that few people succeed at losing weight and keeping it off. That's not helpful or motivating.

There's no doubt that obesity is a chronic condition that can be difficult and complicated to manage in adults. Unfortunately, much of the scientific research is directed toward evaluating why people do not succeed at weight loss. But many *do* succeed. Anne Fletcher described some of them in her previous book *Thin For Life*.

I've spent my career trying to understand what it takes for adults to lose weight and keep it off permanently. For over a decade, my colleagues and I have studied more than six thousand such individuals who make up the National Weight Control Registry, and we have published more than eighteen scientific articles about them. We believe that there is value in learning from those who have been the most successful at weight loss.

Even less is known about how to manage weight problems in maturing children and adolescents. But according to the stories Anne Fletcher presents in *Weight Loss Confidential,* many teens *can* succeed in losing weight. And surprisingly, there are many commonalities in the behaviors and strategies that they use.

Weight Loss Confidential is the first book written from the perspective of teens who used to be overweight and figured out how to get to a healthier weight sensibly. It is not a scientific study, but is instead a real-life look at what has worked. For this reason, it is eye opening and useful. *Weight Loss Confidential* gets at the heart of how the teens do it. And perhaps even more important, why they do it.

Do they eat carrots, do they count calories, do they banish potato chips from the house? What's the role of the parents and how best can they support their overweight children? These are the problems that millions of families face, with very little guidance. This book not only tells the stories of successful teens but describes the strategies that did and did not work. It shows that one size does *not* fit all and refutes the notion that looking for a single solution is the answer for most families. I believe that the strategies described in this book can help many other teens who need and want to succeed. This book provides hope and genuine possibilities to millions of children and adolescents.

— Holly R. Wyatt, M.D.
Center for Human Nutrition,
University of Colorado at Denver
and Health Sciences Center

Weight Loss
Confidential

Introduction

As with all my books, *Weight Loss Confidential* was in my head for years before it came to be. You see, I have a child who became overweight — not just a little, but a lot. By the end of eleventh grade, my oldest son weighed 270 pounds — a weight far too heavy for the well-being of his psyche and his large-boned 6'2" frame.

Wes's weight problem started when he was in sixth grade, and he gained steadily as he turned from the athletic interests of his elementary school days to the sedentary pursuit of high school debate championships. Despite my expertise in the area of weight management, little I said or did made any difference in the habits that led Wes to pack on the pounds. And when he would attempt to cut back, his peers, many of whom could eat whatever they wanted without gaining weight, made fun of him.

I first got the idea for this book from an experience Wes had at a summer academic camp when he was thirteen. While standing in the cafeteria line, he noticed that the kid in front of him was ordering his salad dressing on the side and reaching for a can of diet soda instead of regular. Wes asked him why, since he was so thin. "Oh, yeah?" the boy replied as he pulled out a photo of himself when he was at least 40 pounds heavier. "Everyone in my family eats like a slob, and I didn't want to be like them!"

Wes and the boy proceeded to share weight management tips — something neither one had ever been able to do before with other kids the same age: "Did you know that kids are less likely to make fun of you if you drink Fresca, since the word 'diet' isn't in its name? Did you know that if you dip the tips of your fork in a thick salad dressing instead of dumping all the dressing on top of your salad, you can get the taste without a lot of calories?"

When Wes shared this experience, the realization struck me: *teens typically don't listen to adults—their parents, dietitians, or other health care professionals—but they do listen to each other.* Who better to help teen-agers manage their weight than young people who have done it themselves? Thus, the seeds were sown for this book, but more important, hope was kindled in Wes that he'd eventually be able to slim down. Even though he didn't lose weight until years later, he now says, "I remember thinking, 'If this kid with overweight parents and negative influences could do it, so can I.' Now twenty-one, Wes has kept off 60-plus pounds for three years—a journey he began during his senior year in high school.

What This Book Is — and What It's Not

This book is not a one-size-fits-all prescription for teen weight loss, nor is it intended for teens who want to lose five or ten pounds to look better. Rather, it's a book about healthy weight management for overweight teens and their families—written from the perspective of young people who used to be overweight and who found a variety of sensible means to arrive at a weight that's right for them. (These teens don't necessarily fit society's definition of "thin," but they're healthier and happier than they used to be.) *Weight Loss Confidential* is not only about how the teens got to a just-right weight; it's also about how they stay there.

The teens and their parents share firsthand insights into what works and what doesn't in weight management. I've pored over the latest research studies on the issue and interviewed countless experts, distilling the best of what's out there and putting it all together to come up with sound advice for overweight young people—all the while keeping their best interests in mind from a health and a psychological standpoint. I've also considered the very real concerns that teens face in want-ing to fit in with their peers and in feeling pressured to look like the skinny models and celebrities they see in magazines and on TV—at the same time that they're trying to cope with an environment that encour-ages us all to sit around and eat too much.

In the three years that it's taken me to research and write this book, I've learned that there aren't many well-designed studies on what works for overweight children and teens. In fact, most of the good studies have involved younger children rather than adolescents, and most have in-volved relatively small numbers of young people. And state-of-the-art child obesity treatment programs generally do not have high success rates. Moreover, a recent review of studies on interventions to *prevent* child obesity concluded that many were not effective in preventing weight gain.

With more and more children and teens becoming overweight, it's clear that we need to think about this problem in a new way—perhaps by listening more closely to what young people themselves have to say.

A CONTROVERSIAL SUBJECT

Although I'd been thinking about this book since 1997, I held off on writing it in large part because talk about weight loss for teens even if the teens are truly overweight isn't considered politically correct in some circles. Some experts don't think we should even talk about weight loss for teens. A number of them subscribe to the "fatness (or size) accep-tance" or the "health at every size" philosophy. They suggest putting less emphasis on appearance and on what the scale says and more on health-ful eating and increased physical activity, then accepting the weight that results—even if that means a teen remains overweight.

Although we need to continue to work on changing the stigma as-sociated with being overweight, we can't afford to ignore the very real problems of overweight teens or what the teens who have succeeded at weight loss have to say. In the United States, 1 out of 3 children and adolescents ages two through nineteen is overweight or at risk for being overweight. Indeed, the proportion of children and adolescents who are overweight has tripled in the past three decades, and the numbers continue to rise. Similarly, in the past two decades, weight problems have nearly tripled in Canadian children, and societies that never had weight problems have become part of what's called a global obesity epidemic. As a result, overweight teens face health issues that were virtually unheard-of in young people until recently.

Although some children do outgrow their weight problems, most do not. Several studies suggest that up to 8 out of 10 overweight teens will become obese adults. Both groups are at increased risk for a number of health problems.

When I first became a dietitian, type 2 diabetes, a weight-related health problem, was called adult-onset diabetes because it was seen only in adults. This problem is increasing in young people, particularly in minority teens, including African Americans, Hispanic Americans, and Native Americans. A growing number of kids also are developing conditions such as high blood pressure and high blood cholesterol, both of which increase the risk of heart disease. According to a report in the *New England Journal of Medicine* by renowned child weight expert William Dietz, M.D., Ph.D., about 6 out of 10 overweight children and teens have at least one of these risk factors. More and more children have other weight-related ailments, such as sleep apnea, which is a nighttime breathing problem.

As the teens in this book make clear, our society isn't kind to overweight people. Taylor S. says, "Regardless of how they may appear on the outside and how content they might seem to be, the majority of overweight teens deal with a lot of emotional anguish. It will almost always be hidden, but it's there." After being reduced "to the point of tears" because of teasing, Taylor lost 100 pounds when he was sixteen, and he's kept the weight off for about four years.

ONLY IF IT COMES *FROM THEM*

As the stories of the teens and parents in this book suggest, children of any age should never be given the message that their weight determines their value; they need to be loved without conditions. Over and over, both teens and parents told me that the incentive for arriving at a healthier weight has to come from within the teen, not from the parents.

Taylor S. says, "If a teenager is really concerned with losing weight and has good reason to believe he's overweight, don't tell him he's fine just the way he is. Let him know he's loved unconditionally. However, if he feels he needs to change something about himself, within reason, he has every right to do it and needs to be supported 100 percent."

Tom C.'s mother says, "We should not have told him he looked good when he did not. He eventually resented us for lying to him."

The strategies in *Weight Loss Confidential* are intended for teens who have already shown some interest in changing, not for parents to use to persuade teens that they should change, by saying, in effect, "Look, this is what you need to do." It presents options that teens may choose to attempt or reject—suggestions to be tried on for size.

The good news is that many teens—like Wes, Taylor, and Tom— have found an approach that has worked for them to arrive at and stay at a weight that's right for them. And they've done it without compromising their mental or physical health. I invite you to listen to these teens' stories.

1

Turning Things Around
Moving Beyond Weight Problems

There are millions of reasons to lose weight. Find one, go with it,
stick with it, and believe in yourself. It took years for me to find
the inspiration, but when I finally got it, there was no stopping
me. If you want it enough, you will lose weight.   — **Aaron T.**

> I became motivated to do something about my weight
> because I started to hate looking in the mirror. I wanted more
> confidence, didn't like not being able to wear fashionable
> clothes, and wanted to run faster. Some of my peers made fun
> of me. I stay motivated to keep off 45 pounds by just thinking
> about how much happier I am now.   — **Erin D.**

If you're a teenager who's overweight or the parent of a teen with a
weight problem, you already know that the world can be cruel.
Throughout this book, you'll meet more than a hundred young people
who, like Aaron T. and Erin D., know what overweight teens go through,
because they've been there. Yet all of them have become "masters" of
their weight and moved on to feeling better about themselves. All of
them purposely slimmed down—in sensible ways—and most have
kept the weight off for at least a year. I searched for teens who were not
necessarily thin but who were comfortable with their weight.

This book captures their experiences, wisdom, and success strategies—with the ultimate goal of helping other young people in their
quests to reach a healthy weight. Their stories can not only motivate
others who struggle with their weight but also inspire frustrated mothers and fathers who want to help their overweight teens.

THE POWER OF ROLE MODELS

The teens in *Weight Loss Confidential* are a diverse and inspiring group.

Joyelle T. gained more than 80 pounds in the eighth grade and watched the scale climb to more than 200 pounds. She says, "I was overweight my whole life and felt like an outcast." In tenth grade, she lost 55 pounds, with the help of a weight loss program and through healthy eating and exercise. She doesn't think of her efforts as dieting; instead, she feels that she has changed her lifestyle. Her efforts so motivated her father that he got on the bandwagon and lost more than 100 pounds. Now they're planning a long bike trip together.

Xavier L. was helping his mother clean one of her clients' homes one day when, "for amusement," he got on the scale. After seeing that his weight had climbed to 315 pounds, the fourteen-year-old cried. Today, almost four years later, Xavier is 6'3" — three inches taller than he was then — and weighs 235 pounds.

Robin S. weighed 170 pounds by the time she was nine years old. Her dad is a fitness professional. Her mom told me, "We never expected to have an overweight child." Three years ago, Robin went with her godmother to a Weight Watchers meeting. Now, having slimmed down, thirteen-year-old Robin says, "I'm not in a corner anymore. I've become a much more social person, and I have a lot more friends. I have much more energy and don't put myself down the way I used to."

Rex G. has never let go of his dream to become a star quarterback — a position that typically goes to someone who's lean and quick. Once mockingly dubbed "the fat quarterback" by his football coach, he began his journey to a healthier weight at age fourteen. Now in high school, he stands a good chance of becoming his team's starting quarterback.

Linda Y. was told several years ago that her kidneys would shut down if she didn't lose weight. Beginning at age fourteen, she lost 66 pounds, which enabled her to postpone a kidney transplant for several years. When she finally had the operation, she had reached a healthy weight. Her mother says that before Linda lost weight, she was shy and lacked confidence. "Now," she says, "Linda's a cheerleader and plays varsity volleyball. It's like we have a different child. She has a lot of faith in herself."

McKenzie K. had been "chubby" since she was three or four, according to her mom. At the age of thirteen, McKenzie decided to change her lifestyle. Since then, she has lost 15 pounds and grown about five inches and is now at a healthy weight for her height. When I asked her, "What's the most important thing you did to lose weight?" she told me, "You have to believe in yourself."

McKenzie isn't the only teen who talked about believing in yourself. When I asked thirteen-year-old Summer A. how she found the will to lose 32 pounds, she told me, "I just believed in myself, and I had help from my family and friends." It's not easy for young people who have tried to lose weight and failed to have such confidence. I hope that the triumphs of the teens in this book will bolster other teens' belief in their ability to meet this challenge.

The success stories also may help parents to believe in their children. Psychologist Sylvia Rimm, Ph.D., author of *Rescuing the Emotional Lives of Overweight Children,* interviewed adults who had been overweight during childhood and eventually slimmed down. "The difference for these people," she told me, "was that they had parents who believed in them." The key, she said, was parents sending this clear message to their child: "I know you're going to put this together eventually. I'll be there when you need me." McKenzie K. says, "Parents need to understand that their children can't lose weight alone—kids need to have support and encouragement. It's like running a big race, and you need to cheer them on until they reach the finish line. From then on, you need to continue supporting them."

FINDING THE TEENS

To find out how they lost weight, kept it off, and stayed motivated, I sent 104 teens an eight-page questionnaire. I also interviewed most of them, as well as many of their parents, by phone. A good number of the teens sent me "before" and "after" photos of themselves, which affirmed their remarkable successes. In addition, I asked them what advice they would give other teens who are struggling with their weight. I sent their parents a separate list of questions about what worked and didn't work for their kids and asked them for suggestions to help other parents of overweight young people.

I did my best to reach out to adolescents from all walks of life — teens whose examples would say to others, "I took charge of my weight and my health, and you can do it, too!" They came from thirty-one U.S. states and from Canada. Sixty-three are female and 41 are male. One out of 10 teens in this book is Hispanic, African American, or Native American. The book even includes two sets of sisters who lost weight at the same time.

All were teens or preteens when they lost their weight — the vast majority (7 out of 10) were seventeen or younger when they started slimming down. Thirteen were preteens, most of them age twelve. Currently, 70 of the participants are still in their teens, and most are in the seventh through twelfth grades. The majority of the others are in their early twenties, and more than half of them are in college.* I went out of my way to include this older group because they're living proof that adolescent weight loss can be maintained. For instance, Joe M., now in graduate school, has maintained a 60-pound weight loss for more than ten years. (He's grown five inches, too.) Victoria H. has kept off more than 250 pounds for about seven years.

How did I find all these young people? I reached some by posting announcements on health-related Web sites and by running ads in college newspapers. I said that I was looking for formerly overweight teens who had lost weight in sensible ways and kept it off for at least a year. A

---

*Even though some are now young adults, I refer to them all as "teens," since they were all adolescents (or preteens) when they lost weight.

few big-city newspapers sent teens my way after running my notice as a public service announcement. Other young people were referred to me by commercial weight programs, children's weight programs, summer weight camps, school counselors, and colleagues working in the field. Still others came to me through word of mouth. For instance, one night at my daughter's soccer game, I told another mom about my project. The next week, she called me with the names of three teens her kids knew from our local high school.

THE TEENS THEN AND NOW

When the teens were at their highest weight, the vast majority were overweight — at least 60 of them were very much so. The average weight loss was 58 pounds. Three quarters of the teens lost 30 pounds or more. For some of the most overweight teens, the weight loss was remarkable.

- Fifty-six lost 50 or more pounds.
- Twenty-six lost 75 or more pounds.
- Fourteen lost 100 or more pounds. (Two of them had weight loss surgery.)

On average, they have successfully managed their weight for a little more than three years. Many of the teens have impressive track records.

- For 14 of them, it's been at least five years.
- For 22 of them, it's been at least four years.
- For 42 of them, it's been at least three years.
- For 63 of them, it's been at least two years.

NUMBERS AREN'T EVERYTHING

"Success" can't be measured just by the number of pounds lost, because many teens were still growing when they slimmed down. For some

Choosing Words for Weight

Obese. Fat. Overweight. These words bring pain and shame to those so labeled. "Obese" is a clinical term used to describe someone with excessive body fat tissue who is quite overweight. Because the word "obese" is considered stigmatizing, many weight experts shy away from it, particularly when referring to children and teens. Instead, they tend to use the word "overweight" to describe young people who would be considered medically obese. "At risk for overweight" is a common term for kids whom most people would consider to be overweight or somewhat overweight.

"Fat" has no standard medical definition, but it's commonly used to describe both obese and overweight people. It's preferred by some people who feel that the word "overweight" implies an "ideal" standard, when, in fact, a variety of weights can be healthy for individuals of a particular height.

For lack of a better term, I generally use "overweight" to describe teens who would be considered medically overweight or obese, as does New York University's Sharron Dalton, Ph.D., R.D., in her book *Our Overweight Children*. Terminology aside, the important thing is for each teen to find a weight that's not only healthy for him or her but also realistic and comfortable to maintain.

overweight young people who haven't yet arrived at their adult height, even a relatively small weight loss—or staying at the same weight—is meaningful, since they can essentially "grow into" their weight. Riley M., for instance, is only 10 pounds lighter than his all-time high of 175 pounds, which he hit at age twelve, when he was just 5'5" tall. He is now 165 pounds—a very healthy weight for someone of his height (5'11"). Kristy C., who weighed 140 pounds by the time she was twelve and 5' tall, weighed exactly the same three years later but had grown five inches.

Another reason we can't just look at the numbers when evaluating teen weight loss is that teens who become more athletic may be technically somewhat overweight but are not considered fat, because they're so muscular. That's because muscle weighs more than fat—in other words, a brick-size chunk of muscle weighs more than the same size chunk of fat.

Even more important than reaching a certain number on the scale, the teens I spoke with emphasized, success is about having higher self-esteem, being healthier, having better relationships, sharpening their athletic skills, and more.

9 Myths About Teen Weight Loss

The teens in this book often lost weight against heavy odds. Their experiences challenge conventional assumptions about teen weight loss and the role parents play in it.

Misconception: **Teens who come from an overweight family have little hope of losing weight and keeping it off.**

Facts: Sixty of the 70 teens who answered my question about whether anyone else in their family was overweight said that at least one parent was. Twenty-three of them said that both parents were overweight. Nicole S. is typical. Her mom and dad are overweight. She decided to lose weight at sixteen, when she weighed 293. Although her family didn't think she would do it, they encouraged her to try. Three years later Nicole weighs 145. (She's 5'5".)

Misconception: **Teens who have been overweight since they were young are unlikely to be able to lose weight and keep it off.**

Facts: Many of the teens said that they first became overweight when they were quite young—more than half said it was at age ten or younger. The average age they reported becoming overweight was nine and a half. Fifteen-year-old Sandra D. told me, "I'd always been overweight, even when I was little, and I didn't want to stay that way." Part of her motivation for losing more than 50 pounds was that she was tired of being compared to her nonidentical twin sister, who never had a weight problem. "Now," Sandra says, "we've both grown—and shrunk—to develop a relationship based on who we are instead of on the physical differences that separated us in the past."

Misconception: **Teens who have tried and failed at losing weight many times before don't succeed.**

Facts: Although it certainly isn't physically or psychologically healthy for any teen to go on and off diets repeatedly, the teens in this book provide hope for those who have tried and failed at weight management. When I asked how many times they tried to lose weight before they finally succeeded (counting only the times when they lost at least five to ten pounds), 7 out of 10 indicated that they'd lost and gained multiple times. Forty of them had tried to lose weight three or more times in the past. Sandra D. says, "There were so many times when I felt like trying was pointless, but I finally did it. And if I could do it, then anyone can." Wes G. says, "It took me many tries until I really wanted to lose the weight for *myself* enough to succeed." Kelly D., who tried to lose weight three or four times before succeeding, says that teens need to do some experimenting. "Keep trying new things until you find something that works," she advises.

MISCONCEPTION: **It's best to avoid talking about dieting and weight loss with overweight teens because it's likely to trigger an eating disorder such as bulimia or anorexia nervosa.**

FACTS: The vast majority of teens in this book are living proof that overweight young people can lose weight without developing such an eating disorder. Some studies do suggest that teens who say they diet regularly may be at higher risk for eating disorders than nondieters, particularly when they use restrictive and unhealthy dieting methods. That's why teens need to be educated about how to lose weight in healthy ways and to be shown healthy role models. In fact, Kerri Boutelle, Ph.D., a weight and eating disorders expert at the University of Minnesota, states, "Several studies actually suggest that teaching teens *healthful* methods to control their weight may reduce weight concerns and the risk of subsequent eating disorders."

The truth is, far more teens in our society are overweight than have eating disorders. For instance, the eating disorders bulimia and anorexia nervosa affect no more than 4 to 5 percent of teens. Yet more than one third (34 percent) of twelve- to nineteen-year-olds in the United States are overweight or at risk for being overweight, according to a 2006 report in the *Journal of the American Medical Association.*

James Anderson, M.D., a weight expert at the University of Kentucky who works with teens, sums up the situation this way: "The risk of inducing eating disorders in overweight teens is very low, and the risk from their untreated obesity is much higher."

MISCONCEPTION: **Teens don't want help from their parents in managing their weight.**

FACTS: When I asked the teens what role their families played in their weight management efforts, a strong majority indicated that their families helped them. (Only five teens indicated that their families got in the way.) Both the teens and their parents emphasized that it's important to let it be the teen's decision to slim down if and when he or she is ready. But that doesn't mean kids don't want help and support from their families in their weight management efforts. When John W. was losing 75 pounds, he says, his "family was always supportive and willing to give advice. Now they make healthier meals for the whole family."

MISCONCEPTION: **Teens who say they're "on a diet" invariably have unhealthy eating habits.**

FACTS: Of the teens who said they went on a diet, only some used the word as most people think of it—that is, they actually followed some sort of food plan to help them cut back on calories so they could lose weight. Few said that they followed restrictive diets, and two of those who did went to comprehensive medically supervised programs. When asked to detail their "diets," a good number of teens simply described a healthful way of eating. Aaron T. describes his diet this way: "Having smaller portions, eating the 'right' foods, eating more whole-grain foods, and balancing out what I ate—with the help of a nutritionist." Mia R. says, "I just stopped eating so much and so frequently. I also incorporated more fruits and vegetables in my diet."

Similarly, University of Minnesota researchers Dianne Neumark-Sztainer, Ph.D., R.D., and Mary Story, Ph.D., R.D., who ran discussion groups with more than two hundred seventh through twelfth graders to see how they defined "dieting," learned that more often than not, teens mentioned healthful behaviors when talking about dieting—making comments about things such as eating less fat, more fruits and vegetables, less junk food, and fewer greasy foods. Another University of Minnesota report, on the dieting habits of more than sixteen thousand teens, suggested the same thing for teens who had tried to lose weight using nonextreme measures.

It's the teens who go to extremes with dieting who are at risk for having poor diets and health problems. In yet another study, Dr. Neumark-Sztainer and her coworkers found that teen dieters who used unhealthy strategies such as fasting, skipping meals, smoking cigarettes, and vomiting consumed less of some important vitamins and minerals than did teens who used healthy weight control techniques such as eating fewer sweets, more fruits and vegetables, and fewer high-fat foods. Teen weight expert Thomas Robinson, M.D., of Stanford University says, "I have no problem when teens lower their calorie intake by following a healthy, balanced diet. The goal is to lose weight without compromising nutrition."

MISCONCEPTION: **To lose weight and keep it off, teens need to give up desserts and fatty foods.**

FACTS: The teens talked repeatedly about the importance of not depriving themselves. Many indicated that they eat foods such as ice cream, chocolate, and pizza at least once a week. McKenzie K. says, "If you cut everything out, you'll go crazy."

MISCONCEPTION: **The methods that adults use to lose weight are inappropriate for teens.**

FACTS: A number of experts say that overweight teens shouldn't count fat grams and calories, keep food records, or "work out" the way an adult might, because these things might lead to an unhealthy obsession with weight and food. However, these are the very strategies many of the teens I interviewed used to reach a healthy weight. They don't seem to be obsessed in an unhealthy way. In fact, virtually all of them stressed that the quality of their lives is far better since they slimmed down.

MISCONCEPTION: **Overweight teens shouldn't go on diets because they will just gain the weight back.**

FACTS: Some of the teens I interviewed participated in weight loss programs in which they were placed on "diets" to help them eat less — and they've kept the weight off. Moreover, those who lost weight this way recognize that it's critical to get rid of the "diet mentality." They've shifted from the idea of doing something temporarily to accepting that they have to continue doing many of the things they did to lose weight if they want to keep it off. Katie S. says that she loosely followed a popular diet when she started losing 94 pounds. Today, however, she says, "when people ask me if I went on a diet, I say, 'No, I changed my lifestyle. This is forever. I will never go back to how I used to eat.'" Likewise, Xavier L., who went to Weight Watchers and followed its Points system, which some would consider a diet, advises, "You must change your lifestyle. This is a lifelong process. It isn't about a day, a week, or a month."

It's true that some studies suggest that teens who report going on a lot of diets are heavier than nondieters, but it's hard to know if they really were dieting — that is, if they actually ate few enough calories to lose weight. Eric Stice, Ph.D., a University of Texas researcher who studies teens and dieting, concludes, "I don't think that dieting causes weight gain. On the contrary, I think that effective dieting results in weight loss — and not many dieters cut back on calories long enough to actually lose weight." He adds, "We need to help teens diet effectively and in healthy ways as well as to make changes in food and activity that are not just temporary."

HOW MUCH WEIGHT IS TOO MUCH?

From a health standpoint, what's a healthy weight, and at what weight is a person at risk for developing health problems? Several studies suggest that many teens don't know when they've reached an unhealthy weight — and neither do their parents. In fact, the considerations are different for adults and teens. For adults, the gold standard for defining healthy weight is something called body mass index, or BMI, a number that measures weight in relation to height. When an adult's BMI is 25-plus, health risks increase compared with someone who has a BMI of less than 25; 25 to 29.9 is considered overweight, and 30 or above is obese. (BMI is calculated by dividing weight in pounds by the square of height in inches, then multiplying that number by 703. BMI charts are available in books, at doctors' offices, and on many health-related Web sites.)

For children and teens, the picture is more complicated, because what's considered a healthy weight and normal amount of body fat changes with age and differs in boys and girls. The best way to determine a teen's weight status is to consult a physician and to use special pediatric growth charts developed by the Centers for Disease Control and Prevention for children ages two through nineteen. These charts plot weight according to percentiles for kids of the same age, gender, and height. (The Centers for Disease Control and Prevention provides an interactive computerized BMI calculator that does the work for you. Visit this Web site: http://apps.nccd.cdc.gov/dnpabmi/calculator.aspx.)

BMI and the BMI growth charts are only rough guides for a healthy weight. For instance, some teens fall into the "at risk" category for being overweight because they're muscular, not because they have excessive body fat levels.

It's also important not to go by any single measure of BMI percentile for a child or teen. Rather, BMI percentile should be watched over time to see if a child is staying on track. According to Roman Shypailo, a body composition expert at the Baylor College of Medicine, "The important thing is to watch for significant 'drifting' in a teen's BMI percentile, either up or down." In other words, if there's a sudden large increase or if a teen creeps up by three or four units every year, that's probably cause for concern. But if he or she has been on the same track for years — even if it's somewhat on the high side — there's less reason to worry.

Although it's unwise for kids and their parents to be obsessively calculating BMI and BMI percentile, it's probably a good idea to calculate them periodically, with a physician's help.

TO LOSE WEIGHT OR WAIT IT OUT?

Who should lose weight, and who should "grow into" his or her weight"? A thirteen-year-old girl who weighs 200 pounds will not grow into her weight because that weight is too high to be healthy unless she reaches 6' tall. Recommendations from a committee of experts, published in the medical journal *Pediatrics,* and currently under review, state that weight loss is recommended for overweight teens who have

- a BMI in the 95th percentile or higher.
- a BMI from the 85th up to the 95th percentile if they have medical problems, such as high blood pressure, related to their weight.

However, for teens whose weight problems are less serious — that is, those with a BMI placing them from the 85th up to the 95th per-

BMI Basics

As of this writing, most health care professionals in the United States use the following indicators to define weight problems in teens.

Overweight: The BMI for a teen's age and gender is greater than or equal to the 95th percentile. For instance, a sixteen-year-old girl who's 5'3" and weighs 175 pounds would be in the 97th percentile; a sixteen-year-old boy who's 5'8" and weighs 195 pounds would be in the 97th percentile. *Nearly 9 out of 10 of the teens I interviewed fell into this category at their highest weight; 60 were in or above the 99th percentile before losing weight.**

At risk for overweight: The BMI for a teen's age and gender is anywhere from the 85th percentile up to but not including the 95th percentile. For instance, a sixteen-year-old girl who's 5'3" and weighs 150 pounds would be in the 91st percentile; a sixteen-year-old boy who's 5'8" and weighs 169 pounds would be in the 91st percentile. *Just 7 of the teens I interviewed fell into this category at their highest weight; none were below this category.*

*BMI percentiles were not available for a small number of the teens at their highest weight.

centile and without weight-related medical problems—maintenance is recommended, because they can grow into their weight through physical activity and healthy eating. For young people in this category who are finished growing, gradual weight loss would be appropriate, according to Sarah Barlow, M.D., a member of the committee.

What's a safe rate of slimming down for overweight teens who meet the criteria for weight loss? Dr. Barlow says, "I'm comfortable with a teen losing at a rate of one to two pounds per week. Losing faster than that may mean that the body will start losing too much muscle tissue along with the fat, and that's not healthy. If a teen's hungry all the time, that's another sign that a diet is too strict and weight loss is too fast."

The best way to find out whether an overweight teen should be losing weight or "waiting it out," according to the guidelines, is to check with a physician.

OVERWEIGHT AND ALONE

Although overweight teens have plenty of company in our society, they often feel very alone. John W. says, "Being overweight means you're a constant focal point of harassment because you're supposedly different from everyone else." Sid J. recalls, "People called me names like 'fat ass' and worse." Leigha J. remembers being rudely treated by salesclerks on a regular basis.

Most of the teens indicated that being overweight was a source of great distress in their lives. Tyler D. told me, "I felt inferior. I thought people were laughing at me or talking about me when I was gone." His mother remembers the cruelty and teasing Ty endured at the hands of others—including his three older brothers, none of whom had a weight problem. Even Ty's well-intentioned father, uncles, and coaches needled him, mistakenly thinking that this might motivate him to slim down.

When Ty's baseball coach gave him an award for hitting the most home runs during the season, the coach said, "Ty hits home runs because he's so goddamn slow that he *has* to hit them so he can get around the bases." The coach's remarks so upset Ty's brother—the one who'd teased Ty the most—that he vowed never to taunt his brother again. Instead, he made up his mind to become the coach of Ty's baseball team the next year.

Several of the teens made comments about being sexually harassed when they were overweight. Veronica S. says, "Boys would try to touch my private body parts to see what I would do or say." At least one boy and one girl told me how taunts about their big breasts made them feel bad and drove them to eat even more.

Research suggests that being overweight exacts a psychological toll on young people. Not long ago, a study reported in the *Archives of Pediatrics & Adolescent Medicine,* involving more than 4,700 seventh through twelfth graders, showed that teens who were teased about their weight were significantly more likely to have low self-esteem and serious psychological problems—such as depression and suicidal tendencies—than were their peers who were not teased.

Parents also feel judged because of their child's weight problem. A nutrition colleague once disdainfully said to a friend of mine, "You know, *she* [meaning me] has a child who's overweight."

BUILDING RESISTANCE

Not all the teens I interviewed were tormented because of their weight. Margaret G. says, "I wasn't treated differently when I was overweight—except for very occasional name-calling, which didn't bother me."

Others, like my son Wes, developed a tough shell as a coping mechanism. "If you came across as a tough guy, it seemed like you didn't care what others thought about you or your weight, and it would discourage their comments," he says.

Still others had attributes that seemed to protect them from the taunting. Mike D., who weighed 180 pounds and was 5'8" by the time he was thirteen, says, "I was a pretty funny kid, and I did a lot of sports, so I was treated all right."

Don't Let the World Get You Down
Advice from the Teens

Know that you're above that behavior.

I felt that I was just bigger and better because I wasn't the person that was making fun of another person and trying to make them feel bad. — Molly S.

Realize the people who do that probably have some self-image problem and they're trying to make themselves feel better. Just don't acknowledge it. They're like children, and if they don't get attention, they'll probably stop. — Ben G.

Kids are teasing you about your weight because they're insecure about themselves. Don't let it get to you. — Kristy C.

Don't fight back.

My advice to those who are overweight is "Don't fight back if you are being teased." It's been my experience that the situation only becomes progressively worse if you do. Let them do what they want. When nothing happens, they will eventually leave. — John W.

Just ignore them and don't talk back to them, or it'll be worse. The kids who made fun of me are now trying to help me lose weight and trying to support me. — Summer A.

Believe that it's what's on the inside that matters.

I reminded myself that I was beautiful on the inside and that's what mattered to me. — Jenni O.

I think the main thing an overweight teen can do to cope with teasing is to remember that as long as they love themselves, it doesn't matter what those other kids say. — Mary N.

Turn to your real friends.

To cope with being teased, talk to your friends. They can always make you feel better. More often than not, your friends have been teased about something before, too, and they know how it feels. Although we all know that parents have been there and that they care about us, it's different

when a friend says something nice about you than when your parent does.—
Emily B.

I have great friends who have always been there through thick and thin—
literally.—Sandra D.

Know that weight loss is the best revenge.
Keep your head up. Ignore them. Avoid them. Lose the weight and let that
speak for itself.—Victor F.

Looking good is a great motivator, and losing the weight and being able to
show it off is the best payback. It's great to see the people who called you
names when you were younger and be so much hotter than them. High school
is irrelevant in the grand scheme of things. And the kids who are cruel usually
end up not being able to cope with the real world and continue to be stuck in
high school. It's great to get the last laugh.—Bella S.

Dr. Sylvia Rimm, an author and psychologist, stresses that one of
the best ways for young people to start believing in their ability to succeed at something they want to accomplish is to cultivate strengths in
other areas. This can help shield overweight young people from victim-
ization, as well as protect against eating disorders. In my own family, I'd
like to think that our encouragement and support of Wes's debating
skills and other achievements enabled him to come across to others as a
self-confident person who wasn't picked on because of his size and who
eventually found the strength to take on his weight problem.

What Makes Some Teens Gain but Not Others?

The reasons for becoming overweight involve a complex interplay of
genes and environment. Children come into the world with a genetic
tendency toward a certain shape and weight, but their families' habits
also help determine how they grow and develop. To complicate matters
further, kids may inherit certain tendencies that influence what and how

much they eat. For instance, some may be "programmed" to prefer fatty foods, to eat when they're not hungry, or to be less active.

Children who have overweight parents are more likely to grow up to become overweight adults themselves. Studies suggest that a child's risk of becoming an obese adult is three times greater if one parent is obese and ten times greater if both parents are obese. It's not clear to what extent this risk is the result of unlucky genes or unhealthy habits—certainly it varies from person to person. Whatever the case, there's no question that it's harder for some teens to manage their weight than others. While teens have no control over the genes they inherit, they do have some control over their physical activity and food choices, which are the major factors determining whether most people gain or lose weight.

10 Reasons Why the Teens Gained Weight

From a list of ten possible causes of weight gain—ones experts feel play a role in the obesity epidemic—I asked the teens to check off the five main reasons for their weight gain. At least 75 percent cited the first three causes; each of the other causes was checked by at least 25 percent of the teens. No teen gave just one reason for weight gain; some checked them all. Here's how the reasons rank, according to how often they were checked.

Reason #1: Too much snacking. Molly S. feels that oversnacking was the number one cause of her weight gain. Now, her mother says, "we have nothing very snack food related in the cupboard. Ice cream, cookies, chips, et cetera, have been replaced by fruits."

Reason #2: Portion sizes too large. Erin D. says that her portions were three times larger when she was overweight than they are today. "Now," she says, "when I go to fast-food restaurants, I can't eat a whole value meal. I'm satisfied with a kid's meal."

Reason #3: Not enough exercise. Victor F. was able to lose 50 pounds by exercising four or five times a week, as well as by learning about and practicing good nutrition. Three years later, he still finds time to exercise regularly, even though he's in medical school.

Reason #4: Ate too many sweets and desserts. Wes G., who feels that his number one reason for gaining weight was eating too many sugary foods, says that a major difference for him now is cutting out his nightly "giant bowl of ice cream." (He still eats sweets occasionally.)

Reason #5: Emotional causes (eating when lonely, bored, or sad). Sari M. became overweight when her father left the family. Now when she feels like eating for emotional reasons, she usually goes to a coffee-house, "where the drinks are all fairly low calorie and I can be around people and friends who will hopefully cheer me up."

Reason #6: Spent too much time in front of the TV, computer, and/or video games. Christine F. says that too much TV and computer time were the major culprits in her weight gain. The most important thing she did to lose weight was "*exercise!* It took a while to get motivated, but as soon as there were visible results, I was hooked."

Reason #7: Ate too much fast food. Mick J. told me, "Throughout middle school, I have memories of my mom bringing me a McDonald's dinner every day after school." Now he eats "very little fast food" and says, "I haven't set foot in a McDonald's since 1999."

Reason #8: It runs in my family. With two parents and several other family members who were obese, Victoria H. feels that genetics were the number one cause of her weight problem. She once weighed close to 500 pounds but has been able to lose and keep off at least 250 pounds for about seven years. Although she is still heavier than she'd like to be, Victoria is realistic about her weight goal because of her family history.

Reason #9: Drank too much soda. Ally S. sees this as the number one cause of her weight problem. When asked to describe the most important thing she did to lose weight, she replied, "I stopped drinking soda and sugar beverages. Now I only drink milk and water."

Reason #10: Too many fattening foods served at home. This was on Sandra D.'s list of culprits. She says, "My parents struggle with their own weight, so their examples were not in my best interest. I've lost a lot of weight because of the choices I've made, not because of their influence. However, they do drive me to the gym and buy healthy foods for me."

Why My Son Became Overweight

In my son's case, genetics likely played a role in the development of his weight problem. On both sides of the family, relatives have struggled with their weight, and Wes is built more like these people than the more slender family members. Interestingly, my very lean middle child, who's three and a half years younger than Wes and has a completely different body build, seems to have no weight or food issues. He eats what he wants when he's hungry and stops when he's full. His food choices are not always the greatest, but a lot of the time he just doesn't eat much.

My best guess is that my two sons are "wired" differently biologically. Even when they were little, I noticed differences in their food preferences. For instance, if I told them they could pick out a treat from the candy rack as we were going through the supermarket checkout, Wes would typically go for a gooey high-fat item, while his brother would gravitate toward something low fat, such as licorice. And in restaurants, Wes always seemed to order the highest-fat item on the menu.

It wasn't just bad genetic luck that led to Wes's weight problem. He attributes some of his weight gain during middle school to the two containers of chocolate milk he'd have each day with his school lunch. After school, he'd snack a lot. Even though I tried to keep mostly healthful foods in the house, he says he still found plenty to eat. He'd chow down on half a bag of Chex Mix, skipping the fruit I'd try to get him to have at the same time. Often when we sat down to dinner, he wouldn't eat much, which puzzled me "for a kid his size."

Wes says that when he reached high school, with its open-campus lunch policy, he would "go to the grocery store across the street and get two greasy grilled cheese sandwiches and a huge serving of French fries." Starting in ninth grade, his debate practices and tournaments kept him out a lot at dinnertime and on weekends, which meant a lot of fast-food eating. He now says that he often overate for emotional reasons. Sometimes I would discover quite a pile of candy wrappers under his bed. As a sedentary debater, someone who used the remote control too much, and a kid who would rather die than walk to school, he also became more and more physically inactive as his teen years progressed.

Although I know from firsthand experience that it doesn't help to play the blame game, I've struggled with this, wondering whether his father and I did something to foster our son's weight gain. After all, we tried to offer our kids healthful food choices. We regularly allowed them to have reasonable-size portions of treat foods so they wouldn't feel deprived. And my husband and I couldn't have been better role models for being physically active: we both have exercised faithfully five days a week for our entire married life.

Wes says that part of the problem was that we did everything "right." "Sometimes, doing everything perfectly can backfire," he explains. "There was too much emphasis on healthy eating, and sometimes it seemed like all we had to eat was healthy food. So I felt deprived —like I was missing out on something. The first thing I'd do when I'd go to a friend's house was dig in to the chips." When I pointed out to him that we always had some treats around, he said, "Yeah, but they weren't treats that *I* chose." (He's the first to note that his younger brother seems to have none of these issues.)

The reasons why any person becomes overweight are complex, and there's no simple way to unravel it. Dianne Neumark-Sztainer, Ph.D., R.D., author of *"I'm, Like, SO Fat!" Helping Your Teen Make Healthy Choices About Eating and Exercise in a Weight-Obsessed World*, offers this advice to parents: "As a parent, there is a lot that you can do to help your child maintain a healthy weight. You can serve healthy food at home, help your child be physically active, and role-model healthy eating and activity patterns. But even if you do all the right things, your child still may be overweight. In this situation, you want to avoid blaming yourself or your child and focus on helping him accept his natural body shape. Instead of focusing on weight loss, help your child engage in specific eating and activity behaviors for overall health promotion."

TURNING POINTS FOR THE TEENS

I asked the teens, "What motivated you to do something about your weight once and for all?" For some, there was an epiphany—a precise, dramatic moment or event that changed them forever.

- The deciding moment for Sari M. came one night when she was watching one of those "funniest home video" shows with her mom and her mom's boyfriend. Sari told me, "There was a video clip of a young child, maybe four years old, who was quite pudgy. I made some comment about how, were I the child's mother, I would be ashamed of letting my child get to be that overweight so young. And my mother said, under her breath, 'I am.'" Although I wouldn't recommend this approach for motivating kids to lose weight, her mother's words did prompt Sari to join Weight Watchers. Since then, Sari's mother has apologized profusely for her comment.
- For John W., the turning point was a football injury. He says, "I was sick of being called the fat kid in school, but I found the will to lose weight simply because I had hit rock bottom. After breaking my back in two spots and being diagnosed with postconcussion syndrome, I decided to change my life, because I had nothing else to do. I could no longer play football, or any sports for that matter. The driving force was proving everyone else wrong. I was going to show them that the fat kid could become the skinny kid with muscles."

Generally, though, these dramatic turnaround stories were the exceptions. For virtually all of the teens, a combination of things came together to motivate them to take charge. Sandra D. says, "My weight gave me low self-esteem that eventually hurt my social life. I didn't like going to the mall like most teenage girls, and I was afraid of meeting new people because of their judgment. Lastly, I wanted to be and feel like a healthy person."

6 Reasons Why the Teens Turned Their Weight Situations Around

I did it for my health. To be honest, it floored me that the teens mentioned health reasons for losing weight just as frequently as appearance-related reasons, because over and over I've read that teens are not motivated by health. (It's hard to give up burgers and fries because of that heart attack you might have when you're fifty or sixty.) Nineteen-year-old Taylor S., who once weighed 250 pounds, says, "My main concern was to become healthier, rather than losing weight. I didn't want to die in my forties because of my eating habits. Among the things I stopped drinking and eating were soft drinks, sweets, and any other type of junk food item. I was simply focused on taking care of my body. To my surprise, I began losing weight quickly, and this gave me motivation to continue. Gradually, in a period of one and a half to two years, I got down to my current weight of 150." (He's 5'9".) Angel W., who weighed 240 pounds, says that one of her main motivations for losing weight was high blood pressure. Her 65-pound weight loss brought her blood pressure down to a normal, healthy number — without medication. Vincent J., who weighed 130 pounds when he was about five years old, says, "When I was trying to sleep, it became harder and harder for me to breathe. I was so tired that I'd fall asleep in class. My gym teachers told me that if I didn't lose weight, I would have a heart attack." Today he weighs about 145 pounds and is 5'5".

I wanted to look better. Zack A. says, "I wanted to look hot!" Now, there's honesty for you. Along the same lines, a good number of teens talked about wanting to look good in clothes — or out of them. Lee J. says, "I wanted to wear cute, trendy clothes." The turning point for my son Wes was his first college visit. "It was near the beach, and I wanted to be able to take my shirt off when I wore a swimsuit and look good for girls," he says.

I wanted to feel better about myself. Jenni O. wanted to lose weight because she was depressed and sad, and wanted to feel good about herself. She also wanted to slim down for health and appearance reasons. Ben G. says, "I was sick of being upset and depressed whenever I looked in the mirror or just felt fat."

I wanted to improve my relationships. Many teens told me that they were motivated because they wanted to fit in better with their peers and/or to attract the opposite sex. Mary N. says, "I always had lots of friends, but I could never get a boyfriend. Before I started dating my first serious boyfriend, I remember him telling me about this girl he was obsessed with. He said she was so hot. I asked him what he thought of me, and he said that I was cute. After he broke up with me, I didn't want to be cute anymore. I wanted to be beautiful. I also knew that if I was to date again, I would first need to build up my self-esteem. At that time, I had lost both my first love and all of my self-esteem. I knew that my poor body image had a lot to do with my self-esteem." All of this encouraged Mary to start on the path to losing 50 pounds, which she did more than three years ago.

I was tired of the teasing and ridicule. Thirteen-year-old Jorgey W. says that before she lost more than 100 pounds, "every day, I would come home crying." She remembers being chased around the playground, with her pursuers yelling, "Run, fatso, run," and she was harassed both on the Internet and by phone because of her weight.

My weight held me back. About a quarter of the teens said that one of the main reasons was that their weight kept them from doing things and they wanted to change that. Paula D. says, "I didn't ever feel like doing anything, because I never wanted to go out." Most of the comments about being held back came from kids who wanted to participate or do better in sports or other physical activities. Cole G. says, "I wanted to play sports competitively, and I couldn't with my weight the way it was."

The Readiness Check

Sari M. says, "Unless you want to do something about your weight for good reasons, you probably won't stick with it. If you're happy with the way you look—or you're not unhappy enough with it to do something about it—then let it be. You'll only feel worse about yourself afterward if you don't succeed."

Here are some questions teens can ask themselves to see if they're ready to take steps to reach a healthier weight.

How concerned am I about my weight?

Very concerned _____   Sort of concerned _____   Not very concerned _____

How much do I want to do something about my weight right now?

Very much _____   Sort of _____   Not very much _____

How confident am I that I can do something about my weight?

Very confident _____   Sort of confident _____   Not very confident _____

Do I think I can do something about the things that are getting in my way?

Very much so _____   Maybe _____   Not really _____

How ready am I to change my eating habits?

Very ready _____   Sort of ready _____   Not ready _____

How ready am I to become more physically active?

Very ready _____   Sort of ready _____   Not ready _____

Is my family ready to support me in my efforts?

Very ready _____   Sort of ready _____   Not ready _____

The more answers a teen chooses on the left-hand side of the scales—in the "very" area—the more likely he or she is to be ready to turn things around. Emily B. puts it this way: "It's a matter of thinking about what's more important—eating super-sized French fries or feeling better about yourself. It all comes down to what your choice is." Aaron T. reminds us, "Once the incentive clicks in your mind, you're golden."

Doing It for Yourself

There's one last message from the teens about turning things around, and Aaron T. captures it well: "If you're not motivated internally, then losing weight is going to be tough. I was pushed for about eight years, if not longer, to lose weight. It wasn't until I said, 'I don't like what I am, and I want to change' that I was able to do it."

The teens echoed this sentiment time and again.

- **Victoria H.** says, "It was something I did for myself and no one else."
- **Arahsa L.** says, "It wasn't until I stopped trying to lose for other people that I actually started losing."
- **Tyler D.** explains, "I didn't try to lose weight to gain acceptance. I did it to gain self-respect."
- **Missy S.** says, "I wanted to lose weight for me. I was unhealthy and just wanted a better life."
- **Mick J.** observes, "My desire to finally lose weight was internal. Before that, my mom nagging me about losing weight just made things worse."

In fact, only eleven teens said that one of their motivations for losing was to please someone else.

Athlete Bill S., who has lost and kept off about 100 pounds, says that his coaches encouraged him, and he wanted to please them. However, he adds, "*I* had to want to do it. I didn't want to go through high school and not be known for anything. So I chose to lose weight so I could become a good athlete."

It might be hard for parents to accept, but when teens find the desire to lose weight for themselves, they're more likely to succeed. Zach G.'s mother says, "It's hard when you see your child being hurt. But kids have to make up their own minds. My son really wanted it, and that's why he did it." She adds, "It's a wonderful feeling to have your child take control."

2

Being Realistic
Finding a Just-Right Weight

I'm not going to be a skinny person. I thought I was for a
minute, but I'm not. It's genetics — everyone in my family
has big hips. This is the way I am. If someone doesn't like it,
oh well! As long as I keep maintaining, I'm okay. — **Robin S.**

The teens I interviewed seem to have accepted that it's not reasonable to
strive to look like celebrities and models. They have shown by example
that the best way to start taking control of a weight problem and to set
the stage for success is to be realistic about weight — and to realize that
their self-worth is not determined by what the scale says.

SANDRA D.'S STORY

Sandra D. is a fifteen-year-old who has a good handle on her weight and
her self-image. She told me, "My goal was to lose 50 pounds, and I did
that. Once I got there, I wanted to lose another 15 or 20 pounds, but it's
become less important. I'm content with where I am. I've learned from
experience that it's personality that attracts people so much more than
body type." Sandra is a great role model for being realistic about weight.

She says that she was "never thin" but didn't notice that she was
"different from the average kid" until she was about six. She was an
emotionally strong child, however, and says, "I didn't let my weight hold
me back. In grade school, I took twirling and gymnastics and was even
one of the fastest runners. I got straight A's and was outgoing. Making

33

friends was never a problem—I always surrounded myself with positive people."

Sandra is also self-directed, and as early as fifth grade, she decided all by herself to join Weight Watchers. She now feels that she was too young to manage the program, and she didn't stick with it very long. She also tried the Atkins diet for a short time when her father went on it. Of that experience, she says, "It's not for a sixth grader!"

When she got to middle school, Sandra became a lot less physically active and found herself frequently eating "fast, quick foods on the run," as did the rest of her family. That's when she gained a lot of weight. By the end of eighth grade, when she was approaching the 200-pound mark, her size really started to bother her. As long as she was with her safe circle of friends, she was fine. But because of her weight, when she was in new situations and around new people, she had grown very self-conscious.

Sandra stresses that her parents, who are both overweight, left the decision to do something about it totally up to her.

From an early age, there were a number of differences between Sandra and her nonidentical twin that led to discrepancies in their weight. Sandra explains, "When we were younger, my sister was very hyper and always on the move. Although I was pretty active, too, I was more content than she was to sit and read a book or watch TV. Also, my sister never had the taste buds for the foods I loved—things like ice cream, pizza, and soda. I think that's why we developed different weights and different habits."

Sandra says, "Subconsciously, I felt that everyone was comparing my body to her body. People would say to my sister, 'She's not your twin; she's so much bigger than you.'"

The comparisons led Sandra to do some serious research on her own, right before the end of eighth grade. In a magazine, she'd read about summer weight camps for kids and decided to send for literature and videotapes from different programs. When I asked why she went this route, she told me, "I was already used to going to sleep-away camps, and I thought that if I could go to a weight camp, everyone would be striving for the same goal. I also thought it would be great to go to a camp where I could share clothes with other kids the same size as me." She chose Camp Pocono Trails, in Pennsylvania, because it had Jet Skis. Although it was expensive, her family found the money for Sandra to go for a month.

At the end of the month, Sandra was happy with her loss of 13 pounds. But that was just the beginning for her. She used her initial loss as an incentive to keep losing over the next school year. "I didn't want to waste what my parents had spent. I knew I couldn't fall back to my old habits without gaining, so I just stuck with what I had done at camp."

She proceeded to lose another 37 pounds by paying attention to how many calories she was eating and by going to the gym for one and a half to two hours every other day. She did an aerobic workout on equipment such as the elliptical and rowing machines, as well as weight training. She reduced her weight to 145 pounds, which, give or take a few pounds, is what she still weighs today. (She's 5'3".)

When I asked Sandra why she thinks that she, unlike many kids, was able to keep the momentum going from her camp experience, she replied, "A lot of kids who go to weight camps do it because their parents decide it for them. But *I* took the initiative — *I* was the one who made the decision and wanted it. My parents actually hesitated to send me, because they didn't want to make me feel like I had to do it."

This wasn't a case where the entire family changed to support Sandra. In fact, she went back to an environment where nothing much changed. Her family still ate on the run and didn't pay much attention to what they ate. But they did consistently try to support her in other ways. She says, "I told them what I needed, and they saw that I got it." For instance, when she was losing weight, they paid for her gym membership and drove her there, and now they continue to pay for her membership to an exercise program. To this day, her parents buy healthful food for her, making sure they always have salads and fruits on hand.

Sandra says that compared with how she ate before she lost weight, "now I eat more salad, have smaller portions, eat more fruits and vegetables, drink diet drinks, and drink more water." She adds, "I indulge on occasion. When there's a party or event, I eat whatever everyone else is eating — whether it's chips or cake or ice cream. I just don't eat the bag of chips or the entire cake or a quart of ice cream. Some people ask me how I hold back on Thanksgiving or holidays, and I tell them that I don't. But I don't eat if I'm already full."

Sandra eats fast food about twice a week and typically has one other meal in a sit-down restaurant. However, her choices are different now. "While my family or friends might have burgers and fries," she explains, "I'll have the grilled chicken sandwich and might give my fries away." When she goes to a sit-down restaurant, she says, "I don't eat everything on the dish, and I choose meals on the diet page or get a salad." She still pays attention to calories but doesn't count them obsessively. She says, "I read labels all the time, so I compare products. If one soup has 110 calories per serving and another has 300, I'll choose the lower-calorie one. Or if I notice that a food has an unreasonable number of calories for a small portion, I won't buy it or eat it."

Recognizing that it's not realistic for her to exercise as much as she did when she was losing weight, Sandra has now switched to working out at Curves for about half an hour three to five times a week. (Curves is an exercise program for women.) She keeps herself busy with several part-time jobs and school activities, as well as by participating in the National Honor Society, debate team, mock trial, and school newspaper.

When I asked her how she is able to stick with her eating and exercise habits, she said, "There was a point at which I stopped doing the things I need to do to keep the weight off, but it started to show, and I got back on track. I just didn't want that roller coaster ride." She stays motivated by looking at photographs of herself then and now. "Even though in every picture I'm smiling, I never want to be as unhappy as I was when I was heavier." She adds, "Now I can stand in front of a room full of people and know that they're not judging me because of how I look—they're listening to what I have to say."

As for how she feels about her current weight, Sandra admits that she wouldn't mind losing perhaps another ten to fifteen pounds, but "it's not a top priority. If I don't get there, the world won't end." She concludes, "Many different things make a person worthwhile. If you don't have an ideal-size body, it doesn't mean you're not an ideal person."

FINDING A COMFORTABLE BODY WEIGHT

Most of the teens in this book are no longer overweight. Like Sandra D., many have settled in at a weight that may not be their fantasy weight but is comfortable for them to maintain. Sandra says, "I don't feel that I'm struggling at this weight."

Before they slimmed down, 90 of the teens were at or above the 95th percentile for their age, gender, and height, and 60 of those were at or above the 99th percentile. Here's a summary of where they stand now in terms of their weight.*

- Sixty-two are at a weight considered to be healthy for their age, gender, and height. (Their BMI is below the 85th percentile, or, in the case of those over the age of twenty, their BMI is less than 25.)
- Thirty-one are still technically somewhat overweight, or, as the experts put it, "at risk for overweight." (Their weight is in the 85th through 94th percentiles, or their BMI is in the 25-to-29 range.)
- Eight are still quite overweight. (Their weight is at or above the 95th percentile, or their BMI is 30 or higher.)

*Numbers are from the teens as of the day they completed their questionnaires. Data were available for all but three participants.

No matter what their current weight is, all of the teens are at a weight that makes them healthier and happier than they were before. Note that for the group of eight teens who are still quite overweight, their average weight loss was 90 pounds, and all but two of them lost at least 60 pounds. Xavier L., whose weight dropped from 315 to 235 (he's 6'3"), is still technically in the overweight category. He says, "One man's size 32 is another man's size 38. By this I mean that sometimes people focus on a size that's unrealistic for them and their body."

A heavier weight than is "ideal" for appearance or health is probably realistic for quite a few of the teens, since many of them were very overweight in the past, had been overweight since they were quite young, and/or had at least one overweight parent. If they got down to a much lower weight, they would likely find it a lot harder to maintain. In fact, some teens gained a bit back for that reason. Olivia C., for instance, found that 135 pounds "was too skinny." Today she weighs 150. (She's 5'7".)

Nine out of 10 of the teens accept their current weight.

- Thirty-one agreed with the statement "I'm happy about my weight; it's a good weight for me."
- Sixty-four chose "Although I wouldn't mind losing some more weight, I'm okay with where I am."
- Only 9 said, "I'm not happy with my current weight and would definitely like to lose more."

Like Sandra D., quite a few of the teens would like to lose a bit more weight. But most seem to have made peace with where they are. Sandra says, "I know I can't always be happy with my body all the time. So when I feel bad about myself, I just don't give up. Tomorrow is another day." Wes G. says, "If I'm feeling bad about how I look, I just remember what I used to look like when I was heavier, and anything is better than that."

To Set a Goal Weight or Not?

Sari M. offers some good advice about finding a comfortable weight: "If someone gives you a goal weight, ignore their suggestion. The weight loss program I went to told me that I should weigh 120. But when I got to 130, my body started saying no. However, I pushed it down to 127 or 128 by practically starving myself. I decided that enough was enough and told them I wasn't going to lose anymore." Sari currently weighs 144, which is about 20 pounds less than her all-time highest weight. (She's 5'4".) She says, "I realized that as long as I look good in my clothes and feel happy and good in general, the 'ideal' weight doesn't matter much."

What's a Comfortable Weight?

- It's a weight at which you feel pretty good about yourself, given where you've been. (Yes, you'd like to weigh 120, but since you've been at 180 for a long time, could you live with yourself at 140 or 150?)
- It's a weight that you don't have to starve and exercise fanatically to maintain. (If you got to 125, would you really want to live that way to stay there?)
- It's a weight at which you have no medical problems caused by your weight. In fact, studies show that losing just 5 to 10 percent of your weight — 10 to 20 pounds for a 200-pound person — can make a big difference in your health.

Sari advises other teens to "figure out what your desired weight *range* is and make sure it's healthy." In fact, there's a theory that each person's body has a preset biological weight that it will fight to maintain by causing constant hunger if the person drops well below it. This seems to be the case for many people. However, this number is not necessarily hard and fast. It's more likely a range, which can be quite wide, and people have some control over which area of the range they maintain.

A number of experts I interviewed discourage teens from setting weight goals. They feel that if teens focus on changing eating and activity patterns, the weight should take care of itself. Adolescent eating and weight expert Craig Johnson, Ph.D., director of the Eating Disorders

Gaining — and Growing
What's Normal?

McKenzie K. captures some typical feelings girls have as they adjust to the normal body weight and shape changes that accompany puberty: "I think I'm wide, but people say I'm not. I've got that hip kind of thing going on — you know, when you develop. You have to get used to it. It takes a while, but that's who you are."

As teens who are not overweight shoot up in height, it's healthy for them to gain some weight. According to *Trim Kids* by child weight expert Melinda Sothern, Ph.D., and colleagues, it's normal for a child to gain an average of 3 to 5 pounds for every inch that he or she grows. For girls, the growth spurt usually begins between ages ten and twelve and ends anywhere from age seventeen to nineteen. (Some findings suggest, however, that puberty may be occurring earlier than in the past, particularly among African American girls.) Girls usually grow no more than a few inches after their menstrual period begins, which is usually at age twelve or thirteen.

For boys, the growth spurt typically begins when they're twelve to fourteen, and they usually finish growing at about age twenty, although some grow in stature into their early twenties.

Girls usually have a spurt in weight gain six to nine months before their rapid growth in height, which leads some slightly overweight girls and their parents to worry unnecessarily, as they will slim down when they grow taller. In general, girls gain weight most rapidly — typically about 40 pounds — between ages ten and fourteen, then gain another 10 pounds by age twenty. (Of course, it would not be healthy for a teen who is overweight to gain weight like this.)

For boys, the rapid weight spurt generally occurs at the same time as the height spurt. They gain most rapidly — typically about 45 pounds — between ages twelve and sixteen, then gain another 20 pounds by age twenty.

For girls, other normal changes that occur during puberty and result in the curvier shape of a woman can affect weight, including breast "budding" (which may begin around age ten or even earlier), widening of the hips, narrowing of the waist, and some (normal!) buildup of fat in the belly, backside, and legs.

For boys, changes in body shape include the broadening of shoulders and the growth of muscles.

Program at Laureate Psychiatric Clinic and Hospital in Tulsa, advises, "Rather than pick a weight number ahead of time, teens should see what happens when they eat and exercise reasonably." While some teens will reach a comfortable weight this way, others will settle in at a weight that's still quite heavy.

But teens can find it motivating to set a weight goal. Jane Grace, a registered dietitian who specializes in counseling overweight people, says, "It's unrealistic to avoid talking about weight numbers. Of course weight matters! It's very important to most weight-compromised people. Teenagers aren't any different." Rather than choose a specific number, however, she suggests that teens do what Sari M. did: set a weight range that's realistic, given their body type and shape. Grace might advise a large-framed boy who's 5'10" tall and weighs 250 pounds to set a goal of 190 to 200 pounds. She also thinks it can be helpful to think about a particular clothing size as a goal—for instance, size 34, 36, or 38 pants for a boy or size 11, 12, 13, or 14 for a girl.

It Takes Time

Many of the teens emphasized that it took time to get to their just-right weight. Sandra D. told me, "Sometimes I felt like I couldn't do it in the time frame I wanted to. But I didn't feel sorry for myself. I'd just work harder—not physically, like working out harder in the gym. I'd work harder mentally, telling myself, 'You can do it; you *will* do it.' I just never gave up."

Like Sandra, some of the teens lost their weight over the course of many months or, in some cases, years. Others lost, plateaued for a while, and then lost again, until they arrived at a weight that was comfortable for them. Jeana S., who lost 12 pounds between eighth and tenth grades, then another 10 pounds in college, says, "Changing your body isn't easy. It's a lot like a roller coaster: as long as your coaster is going down more than up, you'll eventually get to where you want to be."

David G., who lost about 55 pounds from the time he was a sopho-

Living with Less than Perfect
Advice from the Teens

Since many of the teens are a bit heavier than they'd like to be, I asked them what advice they'd give to other young people about how to accept a weight that might not be their "dream" weight.

Focus on assets, not flaws. Kristy C. says, "Realize that nobody looks like a supermodel. Even supermodels don't look like supermodels—they're airbrushed and touched up, too. As long as your body is healthy and functional, you need to be okay with it. Don't fret over nitpicky things like cellulite and a few extra inches in the thighs. Try to focus on what you love about yourself instead. Maybe you have great hair or a fabulous smile or bright sparkly eyes or flawless skin. Make a list of ten things you love about yourself and read it when you feel lonely or depressed."

Surround yourself with positive people. Mary N. says, "It doesn't matter how I feel in a swimsuit as long as I surround myself with people who love me and I know aren't judging me."

Recognize how far you've come. Emily B. says, "Think about what you were like before you lost the weight. Accept that you've already done something really hard and that you're in the weight range that's healthy and natural. Be happy that you've come so far and enjoy how much better you feel." Similarly, Taylor S. says, "Do what makes you happy. If you can't seem to lose those few pounds, focus attention on another aspect of your life and return to it later on. Chances are, you'll realize how far you've come and how content you're becoming."

Think about other attractive people who aren't perfect. McKenzie K. says, "Everyone has flaws. Look at Reese Witherspoon, for example. Her bottom jaw sticks out, but she's still really pretty. And Queen Latifah—she's not the skinniest person in Hollywood, but who cares as long as she's happy with herself? It's important to just accept yourself and not dwell on being your dream weight, or you'll miss out on a lot in life."

Accept that life isn't always fair and try to make the best of things. John W. says, "Enjoy who you are, not who you want to be." Molly S. advises, "Not everyone can be a size 2 model. Learn to love your body—after all, you worked hard for it!"

Sandra D. sums it up like this: "No matter what body shape you may have, make sure that you show the person you are inside. Hold your head high and stand tall with confidence in yourself. Your appearance drastically improves when you carry yourself with pride and a smile."

more in high school to his freshman year in college, says, "Losing weight is a journey that needs to be taken one day at a time. That way, you're not too focused on the end result."

COMING TO TERMS WITH BODY IMAGE

Some of the teens still struggle with body image, but they seem to be able to keep things in perspective. Paula D., who weighs 30 pounds less and is two inches taller than when she was heaviest, says, "I realize that my body image issues are probably still with me, and perhaps I may never be able to lose enough weight to be one hundred percent satisfied. But I don't really know how much enough is. Instead, I try to base my satisfaction with my weight on whether I feel good. I want to be at a healthy weight—not anorexic, not overweight. And although I feel like I should probably lose five to ten more pounds, everyone else I know says I'm skinny. So I've learned to believe them over my own probably-biased view." (She's 5'7" and weighs 140 pounds.)

Many young people don't feel good about their bodies, no matter what they weigh. One study by the University of Minnesota's Dianne Neumark-Sztainer, Ph.D., R.D., and fellow researchers, involving more than 4,700 teens, found that close to half of the girls and about a quarter of the boys were not satisfied with their bodies. In addition, a high percentage of girls who were not overweight wanted to weigh less. The heavier the kids were, however, the more unhappy they were with their bodies. Although it's generally believed that African Americans and Hispanics are more accepting of fuller body types and more tolerant of being overweight than are European Americans, there's evidence that kids of all races and ethnicities struggle with how they feel about their bodies.

Reflecting the views of many other young people who think they're heavier than they really are, some of the teens' feelings about their weight don't match their actual weight category. For instance, almost half of the 64 teens who agreed with the statement "Although I wouldn't mind losing some more weight, I'm okay with where I am" were at a weight that would not be considered overweight. On the bright side, some of the teens who agreed with the statement, "I'm happy about my weight; it's a good weight for me" actually had a BMI that would place them in the somewhat overweight category.

Robin S.'s comment at the outset of this chapter about accepting her curvy hips shows she understands that everyone has a unique body shape, no matter what his or her weight. Some people are shaped like a pear, with rounder hips and thighs. Others are shaped more like a square or an apple, having a propensity to be a bit thicker around the middle. Even after losing weight, people tend to have the same basic body shape, but on a smaller scale.

Phantom Fat and Loose Skin

After teens lose weight, it may take some time for them to see themselves as slimmer people. Christine F. says, "I love looking in mirrors and complimenting myself, though I didn't believe myself initially." Based on a study of adult women, body image expert Thomas Cash, Ph.D., author of *The Body Image Workbook,* concluded that people who lose weight commonly experience "phantom fat." The experience is similar to that of a person who loses a leg or a hand but has the sensation that the appendage is still attached.

Katie S., who lost more than 90 pounds when she was eighteen, says, "When I started losing weight, I was not prepared for the loose skin and stretch marks. They were hard for me to deal with. But just recently, I had a tummy tuck, and I'm much happier." (Cosmetic surgery in teens is a very controversial subject. Katie was in her twenties when she decided to have the tummy tuck.) Katie notes, however, that the surgery hasn't changed everything. Although it made a big difference, she says, "I still have stretch marks, and I don't look exactly as I may have expected. But I've come a long way and am very proud of my accomplishments."

In fact, Katie purposely regained about 10 pounds after her surgery to take up the remaining loose skin. "Over time, I've realized that my imperfections are a part of me and they always will be," she says philosophically. "I have to work with myself, though, because it's easy to fall into a perfectionist trap about one's body. What I can improve, I work on to the best of my capabilities. What I can't improve, I have to accept." She adds, "In the past, I felt I had to measure up to others' perceptions of beauty—whether it was peers', family's, or men's perceptions. I feel at peace with myself when *I* am judging my own beauty—not letting myself be influenced by others. Ultimately, I constantly return to the idea that 'perfect' is an illusion and that beauty is in the eye of the beholder."

WHAT SHOULD PARENTS SAY?

Whether a teen is at a healthy weight, overweight, or trying to adjust to a new weight that's healthier but not necessarily thin, parents should not dismiss concerns about weight and having a less than perfect body. The mother of the twins Ashley and Alyssa M. says, "If you try to avoid the issue by telling them they look beautiful, they know what you're doing. It's okay to say things like that once in a while, but don't overdo it."

According to psychologist Kerri Boutelle, Ph.D., a weight and eating disorders expert at the University of Minnesota, "When kids say they feel bad about their appearance, parents often launch into telling them how good they look or how they look better than their friends. But most of the time, all teens want to do is talk about what they're feeling."

Dr. Boutelle says that it's much more effective for parents to validate what teens are feeling rather than to try to talk them out of it. She explains, "A parent might say, 'I can see that this bothers you. I'm sorry that you feel bad about how you look. Is there anything I can do to make you feel better?' Parents can also try to be 'real' with their adolescents, and agree with them that their 'bottom is bigger' than they'd like it to be, but point out their assets as well. This shows that our bodies all have pluses and minuses."

Whatever their size, it's normal for teens to want to look and dress like their friends — something that can be hard for kids who are struggling with their weight. Ashley and Alyssa M.'s mother describes how she went out of her way to make sure the girls had clothes that enabled them to fit in with their peers. She explains, "When the girls were heavy, they wanted tight jeans, like all the other girls were wearing. But when we'd find jeans big enough to fit in the waist, the legs would be too wide. So I'd have the legs tailored so the girls could have fashionable jeans." She adds, "Sometimes you have to accept that they're not going to wear what you think is most flattering for their bodies."

WHEN LOSING WEIGHT GOES TOO FAR

Although I sought out teens who had lost weight sensibly, I decided to include a few formerly overweight young women who initially lost weight in a healthy way, then went on to develop an eating disorder and are now recovered.

The risk of this happening is not high. The Centers for Disease Control and Prevention's William Dietz, M.D., Ph.D., perhaps the most famous child weight expert in the country, reiterates, "Clinicians working in the weight loss business with overweight children and teens just aren't seeing eating disorders in their clients very often." But it does happen occasionally. Here are the experiences of three teens whose weight loss went too far and how they turned things around and got back on track.

Lee J. hit her highest weight of 200 pounds when she was sixteen. She's now 65 pounds lighter, having lost weight on her own — when she was eighteen, after gaining the "freshman fifteen" that college students often pack on when they have free access to campus cafeterias. She slimmed down by cutting back on portions, eating less fat, cutting out regular soda and juice, and exercising a reasonable amount. She says, "I lightened up on the pasta bar and hamburger station, began to fill my plate with salads and lean meats, and joined a college aerobics class." Then, she says, "I let all the compliments that I was receiving go to my

Warning Signs and Risks for Eating Disorders

We don't really know for sure what causes eating disorders, such as anorexia nervosa and bulimia, but experts believe that there are some warning signs and conditions that increase the odds of having such problems. It's important to recognize the signs because, according to the National Institute of Mental Health, the sooner an eating disorder is diagnosed and treated, the better the outcome is likely to be.

Eating disorders may begin with being preoccupied with weight and appearance. Kerri Boutelle told me, "Usually, kids with eating disorders spend a good portion of their day worrying about food, weight, and their body size, while other kids tend to be less obsessive."

The risk of developing an eating disorder increases when teens try to lose weight in unhealthy ways. Experts agree that the more radical the weight loss approach, the more likely it is that an eating disorder will occur. Lucene Wisniewski, Ph.D., director of eating disorders at Laurelwood Hospital and Counseling Centers in Ohio, says, "It's extreme dieting that poses the problem. I get concerned when I see kids with idiosyncratic eating habits—for instance, they decide to take out entire food groups, like dairy products. Or they have very rigid ideas about the right way and the wrong way to eat, with a mindset that there are good foods and bad foods, and they won't ever eat any foods on the bad foods list."

According to the National Eating Disorders Association (NEDA), eating disorders "are most often about much more than food. For some, dieting, bingeing, and purging may begin as a way to cope with painful emotions and to feel in control of one's life." NEDA also points out that depression and anxiety can contribute to eating disorders. According to the American Psychological Association (APA), girls may be at increased risk for eating disorders if they have low self-esteem, have been physically or sexually abused, experienced sexual maturity at an early age (perhaps making them more self-conscious about their bodies), have trouble coping, and/or are perfectionistic. The APA notes, "Daughters of women with eating disorders are at particular risk for developing eating disorders themselves."

Although there are no sure-fire ways to protect a young person from developing an eating disorder, experts say that building self-esteem and cultivating strengths in areas of life that have nothing to do with weight and appearance may be helpful. Similarly, parents and family members should avoid frequent talk about weight, dieting, and appearance.

For more on eating disorders, visit NEDA's Web site: www.edap.org.

head and became anorexic for about two years. The lowest weight I reached by the end of my sophomore year was around 100 pounds." (Lee is 5'9", so her weight at that point could have been life threatening.)

After having severe chest pains and "flutters," Lee was hospitalized for a week for her eating disorder, then had a month of outpatient counseling with a psychologist, whom she saw three times a week. For several more months, she saw a registered dietitian who had expertise working with people with eating disorders. Recovered from her anorexia for four years, Lee is pleased to say, "I finally found a balance of eating and exercise habits that is healthy. I still struggle sometimes with thoughts of restricting food and that I'm fat, but I've learned to cope with life in more practical and healthy ways."

Marie P., who says she's always struggled with her weight, hit her maximum of 175 pounds when she was fourteen and 5'4" tall (which is still her height). When she was a senior in high school, she lost weight with the help of her mother by watching what she ate, learning as much as she could about eating healthfully, and exercising. Before long, though, Marie started working out a lot more and "eating as little as possible." Then, when she went to college, she experienced several major disappointments. "I joined the field hockey team, which was very competitive. I went from being a high school hockey star to sitting on the bench. I was also trying to maintain a long-distance relationship that ultimately ended with my boyfriend breaking up with me. Anorexia resulted because I'd lost all control of my life, and I felt that this was the one thing I could control. I restricted practically everything except for salad and bagels. It lasted for six months, and my lowest weight was 98 pounds."

Marie says that the friends she made in college, as well as a counselor and dietitian with whom she met weekly, helped her recover, as did becoming more religious. "But most of all, I saw the look in family members' faces. One day, I looked in the mirror, saw what they saw, and I was scared." Today, four years later, she weighs 120 pounds and says, "I'm happy with my weight."

Amber M. weighed 297 pounds by the time she was thirteen. She decided to lose weight when she was sixteen because she was tired of being teased and wanted to be popular. She recalls, "One morning I woke up and changed my life. I stopped drinking soda and was determined to do something better for *me!*" She explains, "I did it the old-fashioned way, without surgery or magic drugs." However, once she got down to a healthy weight of about 140 (she's 5'6") by cutting back on fatty foods and walking more, she started using unhealthy means to keep the weight off. "I had anorexia and bulimia, which lasted for almost three years."

With the help of cognitive-behavioral therapy, Amber recovered fully two years ago. "I found a therapist who had experience with eating disorders. She worked with me twice a week for two months, dealing with such intense issues as being molested as a child and shame for being the fat kid in school. We slowly transitioned to weekly, then monthly, visits. As painful as these sessions were, they saved my life."

Today Amber weighs a healthy 145 pounds and says, "I exercise daily, eat a healthy diet with no dietary restrictions, and, most importantly, live each day to teach others exactly how to overcome eating disorders as I did."

Although eating disorders are far more common in females than in males, guys do struggle with these problems. I didn't hear from any young men who had been diagnosed with an eating disorder, but a few expressed concern about sometimes carrying things too far — for instance, by eating too little so that they could get down to a certain weight more quickly. They all reported getting back on a healthy track, however.

SUCCESS ISN'T JUST MEASURED BY THE SCALE

The teens reported that they don't use the scale as their only marker of success. Changes in size also are motivating, as Sandra D. notes: "Notice things like your jeans getting looser or your face looking thinner in photos. I even went down a shoe size!"

But the teens emphasize that there's much more to tracking progress than just going by looks. Improved physical fitness and health are other markers. Sandra says, "Notice that you can do more things — like being less tired after you take part in a fitness test." Victor F. says, "If you're no longer obese or overweight, it's important to acknowledge [the benefits]. You don't have high blood pressure. You aren't stuck in a wheelchair." Bella S. adds, "Be happy that you're now more active and feel better."

For many teens, improvements in relationships are another marker of success. Katie S. says, "Before I lost weight, many people — especially some of my peers — had no regard for my feelings. It still amazes me how much emphasis is placed on being thin and how differently I'm treated now — like all of my worth is in my looks and weight. This is absurd, but it's the way our society is."

As Christine F. points out, losing weight will most certainly improve one's life, but it will not necessarily make all of a teen's problems go away. According to Christine, who dropped 55 pounds about five years ago, "Losing weight did raise my self-confidence a lot, but it didn't make my life perfect. I'm still kind of shy. But I feel confident that the longer I stay healthy and feel good about my body, the more I will continue to grow into my confidence."

Tyler D. concludes, "Everyone has a leveling-out period where they maintain their weight. If you hit this and you're still fatter than you want to be, that should be all right. Look at what you've accomplished and take note of how much healthier, not just thinner, you are compared to before. If you continue to maintain a healthy lifestyle, then what the scale tells you does not really define your health or your worth. Weight is only a number."

3
Letting Teens Take the Lead
How Parents Help (and Don't Help)

> My family helped me by not buying foods that are
> a problem for me. They signed me up at a club and
> helped me be more active. They guided me — they
> opened up the door but wouldn't walk me through it.
> They'd be there and show me things, but ultimately
> it was my decision and in my hands.   **— John B.**

It's tough for overweight teens to arrive and stay at a healthier weight when they don't receive adequate support from the people they're close to. It's especially difficult when others get in their way by nagging them, tempting them, or failing to change the food situations that fostered their weight gain in the first place. Although most caring parents feel for their overweight kids and want to do the right things to support them, the best intentions can backfire. While slimming down is ultimately in the teens' hands, the teens and their parents emphasized the importance of creating an environment that makes the conditions right—both emotionally and physically—for teens to arrive and stay at a healthier weight.

RICHIE C.'S STORY

Each time I talked with Richie C.'s mother, I could hear the concern in her voice. Although she's slim herself, she could feel the pain of her son as he's struggled with his weight. (Richie's father doesn't have a weight problem either, but members of the extended family are overweight.) She told me, "If he needed new shoes, I'd buy them for him. If he had big ears, I'd encourage him to grow his hair over them. But when your kid is fat, you feel like there's nothing you can do." Richie makes it clear, however, that his family *did* do a lot to help him, and their support continues to play a major role in his weight journey. He says, "I have a very good relationship with my parents."

At the age of twelve and a half, Richie began slimming down with the help of Barry Shapiro, M.D., of Briarcliff Manor, New York, who used the Shapedown program as the basis for his approach. (For more on Shapedown, see "Weight Programs Used by the Teens.") When Richie started the program eighteen months ago, he weighed 189 pounds and was just 5'3" tall. Now he weighs 179 pounds and is 5'6".

Richie 's weight problem started when he was five. At that time, he began gaining three pounds a month. By the time he was in fourth grade, he was wearing men's clothing. The family's physician would criticize his parents, and other adults would look at Richie 's mom and say, "How can he be so fat when you're so thin?" This took a tremendous toll on the family and especially on Richie, who was taunted by his peers because of his size.

"When Richie was seven and we'd just come home from the hospital with his new baby brother, Richie didn't know anyone was paying attention to him," his mother remembers, "but I saw him go over and give the baby a kiss and say, 'I hope you don't get fat like me.'"

Richie and his family tried a number of approaches to help him lose weight, including going to Weight Watchers when he was eleven. His mother says, "He refused to go into the meetings. So he sat out in the hallway while I attended them." Richie's parents also tried taking him to gyms to work out, but none would accept a child under the age of sixteen. School sports were out of the question: Richie was too out of shape to make any of the teams.

Without guidance, Richie 's family did what many parents of overweight young people do — they nagged him and tried to restrict his eating. His mother says, "Trying to shame him into shape by telling him how kids will make fun of him and that he'll never get to wear nice clothes just didn't work. When I'd tell him things like 'You should only eat one slice of pizza,' he'd yell, 'Stop calling me fat!' although we never did." The upshot was that Richie just kept gaining weight. "My eating habits were horrible," he says. "But when parents yell at you for eating what you shouldn't, you want to eat more, just to spite them."

The turning point came when Richie saw photos of a family vacation at the beach. When he saw how he looked, he started to cry. "Mom," he said, "I don't want to look like this. Help me." Eventually, his mother came across an ad in the newspaper for the Shapedown program, and they decided to give it a try.

The whole family went to the first meeting. After that, just Richie and his mother attended the weekly meetings. Although Shapedown is usually a group program, Dr. Shapiro used a one-on-one approach with Richie and his mom. The program itself lasted for ten weeks, but they continued to see Dr. Shapiro for ten months because Richie's mom knew how important maintenance is. The entire program, including the maintenance phase, cost $1,700.

Through the program, Richie's mom learned that "telling Richie not to eat something was counterproductive. I'd have to say to myself, 'Don't be the food police.' What worked was having the program educate him about healthy food choices, then asking *him* for suggestions on what to prepare for meals. I stopped telling him what to eat and let him make more of his own choices. Ironically, the less aggressive I was toward his weight and eating choices, the better his response was."

Richie says he liked Shapedown because "it doesn't focus so much on food and exercise; it's more a mental approach. It's how you think of yourself and your image—and whether you want to do this for yourself." His mother says that she liked the program because it is "family based" and focused on health, not appearance. She adds, "It's also based on open communication, and we all had to be part of it. For instance, if we set a goal to exercise for a half hour each day, we both had to do it—

not necessarily the same thing or together. If we met our goals, we each got a reward at the end of the week. Mine might be to spend an hour alone reading. His might be that he got an extra five dollars to spend on something." Why did this help? "It got us away from '*He* has the weight problem, not us.' Instead, the approach said to Richie, 'We're working with you.' Richie's mom also thinks that Richie was able to open up to the physician.

Richie's parents supported him by changing their eating habits as he tried to change his. Richie says, "We used to have a lot of stuff in the house that I wasn't supposed to eat. So we got rid of most of it, and we stopped eating out so often. Now everyone eats the same thing." Richie also learned to communicate better with his parents, telling them how he felt. "I'd say, 'Mom you know I shouldn't have these, so can you please stop bringing them into the house?' And when they'd eat things in front of me that I wasn't supposed to have, I just told them it wasn't fair." (His mom admits that she's a "junk food eater," but unlike Richie, she's able to eat just a little.) The bottom line, according to Richie, is this: "The whole family makes the same efforts I make. I don't feel like I'm the only one."

Richie's mother started reading labels and switched to lower-fat products. She says, "We try not to center family activities around food so much, and we try to be active as a family. That means less eating in restaurants and doing more things like going to the pool and playing family games. We joined a gym together."

All of this has paid off. The boy who couldn't make any team is now on his high school varsity basketball team. Richie also takes tennis lessons, which he pays for out of his own money. For fun, he and his dad play tennis together two or three times week.

As Richie gets older, has more control over his time, and has his own money, his mom admits, "I have less influence over what he eats. But I need to see him as an emerging adult. I'm hoping the changes are all becoming internal now." The mother who once felt powerless concludes, "Setting an example and taking the journey with the child makes him feel loved, supported, and accepted. And *this* makes the parents feel empowered."

How Families Help

Like Richie C., most of the teens told me that they got support from their families in their weight loss efforts. A clear majority said that their families helped them, a much smaller number indicated that their families didn't play much of a role, and only five said that their families made things harder.

In many cases, the family continued to play an important role after the teen lost weight. The most common response in this regard was "They help me," but a close second was "They don't play much of a role." (A good number of the teens are much older now than when they lost weight, and some are living on their own.) Just seven young people said that their families have made it harder for them to manage their weight now.

The teens' parents stressed the importance of encouraging, listening to, and communicating with their teens, as well as complimenting them on making more healthful food choices and on their appearance. McKenzie K.'s mom says, "It's important to be proud of them for trying, even if results are slow to none."

When I asked the teens to describe their families' support both while they were losing and now, their responses centered on these themes:

- They encouraged and praised me.
- They provided material support—for instance, they bought the necessary food or paid for an exercise program.
- They planned and ate healthier meals.
- They joined me in my weight management efforts.

Emily B. says that everyone in her family supported her, particularly her mother, who is not overweight but was willing to accompany her to Weight Watchers meetings for more than a year. Emily says, "It was nice to be at the meetings together, because I didn't feel so self-conscious being the only teenager there. And it was great to be there with the extra support of someone I knew." She notes that her mother also supported her by buying foods to help her with the program and by making healthier meals, something she continues to do. Her mother adds, "And I don't bake so many cookies!"

Some teens inspired their parents to lose weight, too. Jenni O.'s mom says of her daughter, "She's a huge inspiration to me to get in shape."

SUPPORT FROM OUTSIDERS

Support can come from outside the family, too. Some of the teens, such as Eleck F., turned to friends for support. Eleck lost 147 pounds when he was an eighteen-year-old freshman living at college. He found support from a classmate who also was overweight and wanted to lose weight, too. "We were kind of accountability partners," Eleck told me. "We helped each other to make sure we didn't overeat, and we went to the college gym to work out together."

Like Richie C., some of the teens continued to go to a weight pro-gram or receive professional weight counseling after slimming down. In fact, 22 of the 55 teens who lost weight with the help of a program said they still go. For some, that means returning to weight camp in the summer. Others get help on an "as needed" basis. Aaron T., who lost weight with the help of a registered dietitian, continues to see her every four to six weeks "to make sure I don't fall back into any bad habits and that I'm set on the right path."

Some of the teens stressed the importance of group support. Linda Y. and her mother joined Take Off Pounds Sensibly (TOPS). Linda notes, "My mom went to TOPS meetings with me to help herself lose weight, and we still go to meetings together." She says that the group has played an important role in her weight management: "My motivation and encouragement came from the other TOPS members and their faith in me and in one another. TOPS isn't just a place to lose weight. It's a place where friends gather every Thursday night to have a good time and talk about their accomplishments and how to continue to be healthy." (For more on TOPS, see "Weight Programs Used by the Teens.")

What Doesn't Work

When I asked the parents, "What approaches did not work well when your child was trying to lose weight?" an overwhelming response was "getting on teens' backs." The most unhelpful strategies were nagging, preaching, complaining, criticizing, and trying to control food choices. Veronica S.'s mother says, "What didn't work was pushing her and telling her every day that she needed to lose weight and what would happen to her health if she didn't." Eric D.'s mother listed these unproductive strategies: "Getting upset with him every time we ended up having to buy the next-larger-size clothes; telling him what he couldn't order when we went out to dinner; reminding him he was overweight—he already knew that and didn't need to be reminded."

While Emily B. was en route to her maximum weight of 204 pounds, her parents argued constantly about how they should broach the subject. Emily's mother says, "My husband wanted to be much more direct than I and would say things to her like 'Don't order that' or 'Do you need another piece of bread?' But chastising Emily for her food choices or portion sizes just didn't work."

Experts agree that parents should not use food as a reward for kids, nor should they withhold food as a form of punishment. A number of the teens pointed out that such attempts to control food can backfire. Rex G. told me that his parents used to try to control the amount of food he ate during meals by saying, "You're done; you've had enough." This only made Rex eat faster so that he could get more food in before the "cutoff" and led him to sneak food whenever he could get away with it.

Sean C. recalls, "If I came home for dinner and didn't eat much, my parents used to ask, 'What were you eating before dinner?' I'd feel guilty, deny that I'd eaten anything, and then proceed to feel terrible, which only made me want to eat more." Eventually, his parents learned from their mistakes.

The Teens' Advice to Parents

I asked the teens for their advice to parents of overweight teens—what helps and what hurts. Here's what they told me.

- **John W.** says, "Teenagers are rebellious, and the last person they want to listen to is a disciplinarian parent laying down the law about 'this is why you need to lose weight.' If you talk to teenagers on a friendly level, a lot more about the problem will be revealed."

- **McKenzie K.** advises, "Don't tell teens they're fat or lazy. They probably hear that enough from peers, and things like that bring down their self-esteem. You can't be motivated to do something if you don't feel good about yourself."

- **Aaron T.** says, "Don't make overweight kids feel singled out at the dinner table, like by having meals that are different from everyone else's. Use your child as an opportunity for the whole family to eat better. Also, especially in the early stages, don't make it widely known that your child is trying to lose weight. Let people notice it on him or her or hear it from your child's mouth. It's not something that needs to be broadcast to the world. It can be a very stressful time, especially if the weight is not coming off right away. So cut your child some slack."

- **Emily B.** notes, "Be supportive of their choices. And if they mess up, don't get angry. Help them learn how to handle it next time. Make sure to talk to teens about what they're going through, because it's hard, and parents are easier to talk to about weight than friends are most of the time."

BACKING OFF

When I asked the parents, "What *did* work?" and "What advice do you have for other parents of overweight kids?" many stressed that backing off is an important strategy. Joyelle T.'s parents explain, "We let Joyelle make her own choices. She knew what was best for her. We never said what she should or shouldn't eat or do." Sean C.'s dad adds, "The less-is-more approach is what worked. By not criticizing or badgering him, we left the ultimate decision up to him. If you have a teenager, you have to be realistic. You cannot and will not control them."

Sid J. says, "I hate being told to do something, and that includes being told what to eat and not eat. *I* prefer to have control over my eating."

Sometimes teens give their parents conflicting messages about whether they want them involved or not. Sean C.'s father recalls that before a party, Sean asked for a reminder if he seemed to be eating too much. When his dad gave him a subtle sign that no one else could see, "Sean was mortified," his father told me. Other times, when Sean and his dad went to a restaurant, he'd ask his dad, "What's good for me?" If his dad said something like "Try the fish," Sean would look at him as though he had "just dumped five inches of rain on the parade." His father said, "Finally, I realized that I could only do so much and that Sean would have to take responsibility. If I, in any way, indicated disappointment or put pressure on him, it was disaster."

When Sean was twelve and a half, he became interested in girls and was sick of being teased about his weight. This prompted him to ask his parents for a treadmill, which they bought. On his own, with little input from his mom and dad, he proceeded to lose 40-plus pounds, which he's kept off for about seven years. Sean says, "Continually asking my dad what I should order—which usually resulted in my ordering a hamburger anyway—eventually turned into my remembering what he said. Those messages finally sunk in." Sean believes that this happened because his father's advice in these situations "was always nonjudgmental." He concludes, "When my parents gave me the tools to succeed but didn't necessarily implore me to use them, that's the time when it inspired the most self-reflection. When I was left to my own devices, I decided it was in my best interest to make the changes."

THE IMPORTANCE OF OWNERSHIP

Sid J.'s mother was one of several parents who emphasized the importance of encouraging kids to have "ownership" of the weight management process. She explains, "If a child is constantly relying on someone who says, 'Don't eat this' or 'Don't eat that,' it doesn't work. At some point, he has to begin to own his own eating habits. This happens when you give them choices." For example, she would ask Sid, "Do you want me to remind you about how much you're eating or not?" If he said he did, they used cues so he wouldn't be embarrassed. The signal might be for her to touch her ear or to say, "Oh, I'm so full." She adds, "It worked better if I could also catch his eye. I always did it with a smile, though, so he'd know I wasn't angry."

Part of ownership is, as Sid's mother says, realizing that "no change will occur unless the child wants it." Emily B.'s mother confirms this point: "Let the child decide. No program will work if the child is not invested in the process and outcome."

READINESS IS EVERYTHING

Pushing teens to lose weight before they're ready to make a commitment to change their eating and exercise habits can set them up for failure, bruise their self-esteem, and discourage future weight loss attempts. I sometimes called my son's pediatrician to talk about his accelerating weight the day before a routine checkup. The doctor would say, "If it's a concern for Wes, we'll address it. If not, we'll leave it alone." Some peo-

How *Not* to Talk to a Teen

Steven Berg-Smith, M.S., coauthor of a study on how to motivate teens to improve their diets and a health psychologist who owns the California-based company A.I.M. for Change, urges parents to avoid the following pitfalls that can generate resistance and entrench a teen in a no-change position.

- Using a judgmental or confrontational approach
- Trying to "talk sense" into them
- Using restrictive language ("you have to"; "you can't"; "you need to"; "you should")
- Trying to be too helpful and asking too many questions
- Patronizing, dismissing, or minimizing feelings

Mr. Berg-Smith points out that when a teen offers a hopeful sign that he or she might be interested in changing, it's best to use restraint, not to pounce. For instance, if a teen says, "My pants are too tight; I look really gross," don't respond with "Let's sign you up for the YMCA weight program." Rather, say, "Do you want to talk about it?" (My son Wes says, "Let them know you're willing to talk, then back off.") When you see signs that a teen is trying to change, it helps to focus on successes and efforts versus what's not happening. For instance, if a teen comes home from school and goes for a long walk, then sits down and eats a bowlful of buttered popcorn, say something positive about the fact that she took a walk and restrain yourself from mentioning the popcorn.

Mr. Berg-Smith adds, "Teens are more motivated by what they hear themselves say than by what someone else tells them, so let *them* make their own arguments for lifestyle change and ways of achieving it." So if a teen expresses an interest in starting an exercise program, rather than jump in with all of your ideas about what type of exercise is best or how to start out, ask what types of exercise he has considered and how he thinks he might go about getting started.

ple might argue that this approach is passive. But Wes says, "Pressure to lose weight from outside forces, like parents, coaches, and health teachers, only led to guilt. And that just made me eat more."

Although I didn't try to impose any weight loss schemes on Wes, he says that my constant reminders—such as "Don't sit down with the whole box of crackers; put some in a bowl" and "Why don't you have a piece of fruit with those chips?"—only served to remind him of all the things he *wasn't* doing. That just made him feel guilty, which in turn made him want to eat more. Wes says, "Once you tell kids something like this, they know it. When you kept reminding me all the time, it just reminded me that I had a weight problem." In the end, Wes says, "all the things that you taught me about losing weight were the things I ended up using when I finally did it. But it was a matter of maturity and being ready."

GENTLE NUDGING

Gentle advice may help a teen, but it's best when offered in response to a request or a sign that the teen actually wants help. Emily B.'s mother got such a sign one day when they went shopping together and she could see that her daughter was unhappy about how she looked. That night, she says, "when I went to tuck Emily into bed, I said, 'I noticed, sweetheart, that today you didn't seem happy about how clothes were fitting you. Is that right?'" Emily said yes. Then her mother suggested that maybe Emily would be happier if she lost some weight, mentioned an adult friend who'd had success with Weight Watchers, and asked Emily if that was something she'd like to look into. She agreed, and her mom said, "Great. I'll make an appointment. If you don't feel comfortable, we won't continue. But let's give it a try."

Emily says that when her mother first mentioned trying Weight Watchers, she was upset because she "didn't like being told what to do." She adds, "But my mom approached me from my perspective, noticing that I didn't seem very comfortable in my clothes. And she was sensitive about taking me to a weight loss program, which made it easier. Once I lost weight the first week, I realized I could do it, that it was worth it, that I felt a lot better, and that it wasn't just for my mom." Emily's mother attended weekly meetings with her for more than a year, and Emily lost about 60 pounds while growing another inch.

THE IMPORTANCE OF UNCONDITIONAL LOVE

Quite a few of the parents emphasized that unconditional love is critical, no matter what happens to a teen's weight. Richie C.'s mother advises, "Don't criticize children who are overweight — they get enough rejection in the outside world. Let them know they are loved and accepted at home." Sean C.'s dad adds, "Do not dwell on overweightness as a problem or concern. Overweight children know how you feel. Keep your child unconditionally loved and hope — hope — that he or she eventually sees it's in their interest to lose weight."

None of this is to say that parents should throw up their hands and abandon all efforts to help their overweight teens arrive at a healthier weight. Eric D.'s mother, who emphasized unconditional love and who found that trying to restrict what Eric ate didn't work, says, "Giving up on trying to help Eric with his weight loss when he was content with the computer and movies on TV wasn't the solution either."

BEING A ROLE MODEL

Richie C.'s mother told me, "We sent the wrong message by telling Richie to go outside and be active while we, as his parents, were living a sedentary lifestyle. We had to practice what we preached."

Indeed, when I asked the teens' parents for their advice to other parents of overweight children, the number one response was "Be a role model." Similarly, when I asked them how parents can avoid having their kids gain excessive weight, their top response was to be living examples of healthy eating and exercise habits.

When asked whether their habits have changed since their teens lost weight, many said yes. Others said that they had previously made changes in their eating and exercise habits, which spurred their teens to take action. Rebecca M.'s dad started losing weight before she did. When it became noticeable, she asked how he did it. He says, "I never talked to my daughter about her weight and never tried to impose any approach. On her own, she decided to lose weight, and I noticed that she started to change her eating habits just as I had done. Once she indicated that she wanted to lose weight, I helped her by indicating how she could make better food choices. There was nothing in particular that I did to support her other than to let her know that I could tell that she was losing weight and that she was doing a good job on her new 'food program.'"

He adds, "When I was losing weight, I stopped going to McDonald's and other fast-food places and told my daughter that I couldn't find anything on the menu that was good for me. However, if that was where she wanted to eat, I would take her there, and then we'd go to a different place for my food. It wasn't long before she also gave up on fast food. When I prepared food at home, I'd make something for me and ask Rebecca what she wanted. Again, it didn't take very long before we both ate the same thing."

Some of the teens told me that their parents' examples set the stage for them. Kristy C. says, "I never would have started exercising if my mom hadn't been working out for my entire life. She makes time every day to exercise, and she's a very busy woman, what with raising a family and advancing in her career. So I knew I could fit it in my schedule, too." Aaron T. says, "The best thing I had was my dad, who lost weight and now is more 'built' than most of my friends. It was great to have my dad to look up to—as someone who works out and eats healthy."

Although it can be hard for families with busy schedules to sit down and eat together, meals provide an opportunity for teens to see their parents eating healthfully and to get an idea of what a well-balanced meal is. Emily B.'s mother says, "Eating together is a chance to communicate with each other and offers an opportunity to get to know each other in a way that other activities don't allow." There's some evidence that family meals lead to more healthful eating, too.

One large study reported in the *Archives of Family Medicine* showed that the more often families ate dinner together, the more healthful were the dietary patterns of nine- to fourteen-year-olds. Other studies have revealed that parents who eat fruits and vegetables have kids who do the same.

Some of the families explained how they involved everyone in the effort to eat more healthfully. McKenzie K.'s mother says, "We discussed lifestyle changes with the whole family, rather than focusing on one individual. We talked about portion control and healthy, balanced choices, but we discouraged any talk of 'diet.' We started the whole family reading labels to distinguish healthy food from junk food. The message was never 'don't have something'; it was comparing foods to see which one was healthiest."

Teens also need to see their parents as role models for healthy amounts of physical activity. Often parents who exercise do it apart from the family, and the only time kids see their parents may be in front of the TV in the evening. Jamie L.'s mother says that one of the best approaches when she was trying to support Jamie in her weight management efforts was "buying an annual family fitness club membership and joining Jamie at the club as much as possible." She adds, "Buying the membership has forced three out of four of our family members to go to the club frequently. Our mental and emotional attitudes have improved while working out."

Finally, it's important for parents to avoid modeling unhealthy dieting practices. One teen told me, "I'd heard about the Atkins diet from my mom because she'd been on it all the time, and I was interested in seeing how it would work for me. So I tried it." At the same time, this girl also started doing workout videos, on top of being on the high school tennis team. She found that "all that exercising and no carbohydrates was really hard on my body. At tennis matches, I felt sluggish and out of energy." Eventually, her friends convinced her that it would be healthier if she started eating carbs again.

CHANGING THE FOOD CLIMATE

One of the strongest messages from the parents and teens alike was that families need to keep healthful foods around the house and avoid having many unhealthful ones. Mary N. says, "Parents need to understand that having tons of junk food around is practically sabotage."

Kristen F. told me, "Before, there was always candy, cookies, chips, and sugar drinks in the house. Now my friends come over and say, 'You don't have any snack foods!'" Her mom explains how the family has changed: "We didn't have fresh fruits because I wouldn't spend the extra money for things like fresh strawberries or blueberries. Now I just buy them. We also switched to whole-wheat bread and skim milk. Once in a while, we buy sweets, but not nearly as many as we did before." She adds that when she actually "put a pencil" to a cost comparison, "even the most expensive fruits were less money than the processed candies, cookies, and chips."

Kristen says that this change has taken the pressure off. "If tempting foods are around, you feel like your family's not supporting your ambitions. When you're home, you want to relax and not have to worry about being tempted."

Zach G.'s mother says, "If you want teens to eat healthy foods like fruits and vegetables, you have to have that stuff easily accessible." She keeps foods such as cut-up carrots and melon on hand. When she grills chicken or shrimp, she makes a lot at one time, so it's ready if Zach wants to snack. She also makes her own low-calorie pita pizzas and keeps them in the freezer so that Zach can easily pop one in the oven. She says, "Yes, it's work for the parents. But if Zach overeats, I know it will be these things, because it's what we have available."

Busy parents have to figure out how many changes they can handle and how much preparation time they can spare. Richie C.'s mother found that the changes their physician suggested in her cooking were just too much for her. "He gave me low-carb recipes that were hard to make and had ingredients that my family won't eat. It made me feel like I had the full responsibility and like it would be my fault if he gained weight. I started seeing it as a chore, which sometimes made me feel angry and think things like 'Look what I've got to do because of you.'"

Finally, she gave up on the new recipes and made changes she was comfortable with. "I focused on portion control and bringing the right things into the house. I read labels and tried to be careful with fat. We used smaller plates, so portions looked bigger. I made it a practice to serve food from the stove, not family style. If anyone wants more, they can ask for it." At one point, she found herself cooking different meals for different people in the family. "I caught myself and told them, 'This isn't a restaurant, where everyone gets to order what they want.'" Now everyone is served the same foods at meals.

WHEN FAMILIES DON'T CHANGE

Although many of the parents said that their eating habits have changed for the better since their teens started slimming down, more than half of the teens reported that they eat differently than the rest of their families — most of them more healthfully. Some said that they're more aware of portion size and the nutritional value of foods. Others said that they eat less meat; drink less regular soda; have less fat, carbs, or sweets; or dine out less often than other family members.

Mia R. finds it difficult to deal with her family's traditional Latino food habits. She explains, "They expected me to get on a diet and lose weight while they had delicious Spanish food. Everyone in my family eats rice and beans, which are okay if you eat reasonable portions. But everything we eat is either sautéed, fried, or accompanied by rice. Like for breakfast, we'll eat fried plantains with fried cheese, and we can have that as dinner, too."

I asked the teens how they cope when other family members are overeaters. Aaron T. says, "It's very hard but not impossible. My mom is like Betty Crocker in the kitchen—I could be 400 pounds. The best way to handle it is to do what my dad and I do: spend as little time as possible in the kitchen and never do work in the kitchen. At dinner, I take a plate and whatever is on that plate is all I'll eat—no seconds." Mary N. says, "When I see my family overeating, I usually try to do something that will take my mind off eating. I play Nintendo, read, or work out."

Some of the teens whose families overeat view them as examples of how they don't want to behave and use this to fuel their own determination. Taylor S. says, "I use my family members as a motivation to stay on track." Ben G. thinks observing others' habits can be an educational experience. He says, "Try to see what you could do differently. Use it as a learning tool rather than an obstacle."

Other teens have seen a degree of change in their families. Victor F. says, "I come from a family that overeats. However, over time we've learned about moderation. Overeating still occurs but with healthier food. For instance, instead of a large bowl of rice, it will be a large bowl of vegetables. Instead of fried chicken, it will be grilled chicken."

DEALING WITH "FOOD PUSHERS" AND SKINNY FRIENDS

Some of the teens told me that they often had to cope with relatives or friends who insisted on trying to get them to eat foods they wanted to avoid. Jon M. says, "As a young man, you're supposed to eat everything. I just say, 'No thanks.'" Thirteen-year-old Sullivan A. says, "'No thanks.' If they don't listen to me, I just stand up and walk away."

Not all of the teens are so adamant; some take a little of the food that's being offered. Others might say that they don't like a particular food or they're allergic to it. When Jack F. is pressed to eat something he prefers not to, he explains what he's accomplished and says he doesn't want to gain the weight back.

Tyler D. offers some preemptive advice: "Once people know you're trying to lose weight, they subconsciously try to sabotage you by saying things like 'Oh, you don't need to lose weight. Here, have a cookie.' I think it's better to tell others you're trying to be healthier instead of trying to lose weight."

One of my son's greatest challenges was being with friends who seemed to be able to pack away any type of food in any amount without gaining weight. Aaron T. says, "My best friend can make ice cream disappear. I spent a whole summer watching him down Ben & Jerry's ice cream while I stood there and said, 'Nothing for me, thank you.' It's not easy knowing that some people can eat whatever they want, but hey, life is not fair. I rationalized it by saying I saved money, and on free-cone day, I conceded and had ice cream."

Some of the teens told me that they've simply grown to accept that everyone's different and that not being able to eat the way their friends do is just the way it is. Taylor S. finds this easier to deal with when he concentrates on what he has that his friends don't, such as his musical ability or his creativity. And several of the teens said that they remind themselves that thin kids who don't have to worry about what they eat are not necessarily healthy. Kristy C. says, "They're probably clogging their arteries now and will have problems in the future."

WALKING A FINE LINE

The teens and their parents reported that haranguing overweight kids about their weight and restricting foods doesn't work. But they, like many experts in the field, also said that families should avoid bringing unhealthful foods into the home. So how do families create a healthy food environment without having their overweight kids feel deprived?

Kristen F.'s mom admits, "It's a struggle." Often, she would bring home sweets, because *she* loves them, and hide them — but Kristen always found them. Then Kristen came up with a plan. She'd have her mother buy something like half a bundt cake (not a whole one), and Kristen would cover it up on the counter. Her mother says, "That way

Kristen had control of it." She adds that the family also kept plenty of healthful choices around, such as fruits and vegetables. Kristen says, "I might wind up eating the cake and some fruit together, but doing this did help me eat less of the unhealthy food than if I'd had it by itself."

Researcher Leann Birch, Ph.D., of Penn State University has conducted a number of studies suggesting that at least in young children, restricting highly palatable foods may lead to increased preference for them. Nevertheless, she believes that overall the food climate in homes should focus on healthy foods and limit high-calorie items. She says, "What really gets to kids is when tempting foods are in the house but they feel they can't have them. The goal is to place kids in an environment that sets them up to make healthy choices. If ice cream is a problem for a teen, then don't keep half-gallons in the house; instead, go out for some."

That's exactly what Kristen and her mother sometimes did when Kristen felt discouraged and said things like "I can't eat foods normal teenagers eat." Occasionally, her mother would respond, "So let's just go and have some ice cream." They'd get a mini-sundae and that would help Kristen feel better. "She'd see that she could have a small portion and still be okay with her weight," her mom says. Sometimes they'd do something not related to food to lift her spirits. For instance, they'd drive to Walgreens just to read the funny greeting cards. "Soon," Kristen says, "I'd be laughing so hard, I'd forget about food."

Like Kristen's mother, Zach G.'s mom enjoys sweets and occasionally buys them for herself. But if she buys cookies, Zach will keep eating them until they're gone. Here's how he handles it: "My mom buys stuff sometimes, but I tell her to hide it." His mother explains, "Hiding the food is *Zach's* suggestion. But when he tells me not to buy something, I stop buying it." She also made it clear that most of the choices at home are healthful ones and that, within those, Zach makes his own decisions about what he eats and how much.

Ultimately, the teens know they have a stake in having a healthy food climate, and as these examples show, the impetus comes from them, not just their parents. Zach, who lost weight at a summer weight camp, says, "When I came home, I told my mom I wanted to keep doing the stuff I learned at camp—like eating healthy meals—and she supported that."

Sean C. concludes, "Parents have to firmly and silently set the tone by having healthy foods around the house. Let the kid go out and eat junk food, but don't make him feel bad about it. In the end, he has to learn through trial and error. If parents are not overbearing, the kid will eventually see that it's not in his self-interest to be overweight. It really comes down to the child accepting the cards he was dealt and not feeling sorry for himself. That epiphany comes from inside, not from being forced on you."

4
Discovering What Works
Individualizing Weight Loss Strategies

> Find a diet and exercise plan that's right for you. If you enjoy the foods and activities, you're more likely to stick to a healthy lifestyle. — **Ally S.**

The stories of the teens reveal that, in the end, losing weight is a highly individual process. Ally S.'s words capture what I learned from their responses: there is no single program or diet that works for everyone, no magic bullet. To arrive at a healthier weight, teens have to do what's right for them, as individuals. More than four years ago, Ally began losing the 56 pounds that she eventually shed by giving up regular soda, cutting back on junk food, and walking on a treadmill while she watched TV. Other teens chose very different routes to a healthier weight.

LONERS VS. PROGRAM TEENS

From summer weight camps to one-on-one help from a dietitian to coming up with their own creative plans, the teens' methods represent a potpourri of sensible approaches for getting to a healthy weight. The teens were split almost fifty-fifty between loners and program people: 49 of them slimmed down on their own, while 52 did it with the help of a program or health care professional. Another 3 lost some weight on their own, then went to a program.

Of the program people, some went to well-known, nationally available programs designed for children and teens, while others went to smaller, one-of-a-kind programs run by an individual, hospital, or clinic. Others went to programs primarily designed for adults. (A description of the specific programs that referred young people for this book can be found in "Weight Programs Used by the Teens.")

- Seventeen went to summer overnight camps designed to help young people lose weight.
- Eleven went to weight management programs designed for children and teens.
- Twenty-one went to weight programs designed primarily for adults. Of these, 12 went to commercial programs, 3 went to a nonprofit program, 2 went to an intensive medically supervised program, 3 went to a program that focuses mainly on exercise, and 1 went to a program developed by a registered dietitian.
- Four had individual counseling from registered dietitians with expertise in weight management.
- Two went to respected programs for obesity surgery.

The teens' experiences demonstrate that it's critical that they decide how (and if) they want to arrive at a healthier weight. Kyle B. advises parents, "Don't plan a teen's diet for him or her. If he wants to try the grapefruit diet and the parent spends all day researching the South Beach Diet and persuades the teen to try that, chances are the kid won't stick with it. Let your child learn what works and what doesn't on his own." While I'm not endorsing these diets and believe that teens need some guidance for healthy weight loss, Kyle's point is well taken.

Scattered throughout this chapter are stories of how different teens found their own way to a healthier weight. None of these approaches is the right way or the wrong way to slim down. Each has its pros and cons.

Slimming Strategies

Strategy	Number of Teens Who Used Strategy
I exercised more.	86
I cut back on foods high in fat.	48
I went on a diet.	47
I stopped eating certain foods completely.	42
I counted calories.	29
I continued to eat all foods, just ate less of them.	26
I skipped meals.	14
I used a liquid supplement or protein/energy bar in place of meals.	11
I used diet pills or weight loss medications.	5
I fasted (went without eating for a day or more).	3
I smoked cigarettes.	1
I made myself vomit.	0
I took laxatives.	0

SLIMMING STRATEGIES USED BY THE TEENS

I wanted to know exactly what strategies (both sensible and questionable) the teens used to lose weight and which ones were most common. As the following chart shows, the vast majority of the strategies were sensible—eating fewer fatty foods, getting more physical activity, watching calories, and cutting back on food in general. Most of the teens used a combination of strategies.

What's most striking is the preponderance of healthy strategies the teens used to arrive at a healthier weight. Exercise (or generally becoming more physically active) was the front-runner. My guess is that most people would think that diet would rank first, so it may come as a surprise that exercise was the most frequently mentioned strategy, far ahead of all the others used by the teens. When asked what types of exercise they did while losing, the teens gave many different responses, but the most common ones were running, walking, and lifting weights.

Cutting back on fatty foods and "going on a diet" were neck and neck for second place—both mentioned by close to half of the teens. Although 47 of them indicated that they went on a diet, there was a lot of variation in what this meant. In a number of cases, it simply signified healthy eating. Of those who actually used some sort of diet, the vast majority used sensible, healthy approaches.

Doing the Math:
What's a Safe and Healthy Calorie Level?

To go from being overweight to a healthy weight, teens, like the rest of us, need to eat fewer calories than their bodies use each day, or they need to increase their physical activity so they burn up more calories than they eat. The vast majority of the teens learned that the best way to lose weight is to do both.

Calories are not nutrients. Rather, calories measure the energy that we get from eating three types of nutrients in foods: carbohydrate, protein, and fat. (The other nutrients—vitamins, minerals, and water—provide no calories.) Carbohydrates and protein provide about 4 calories per gram, while fat provides about 9 calories per gram. Alcohol, which is not a nutrient, provides about 7 calories per gram. (A gram is about one thirtieth of an ounce.)

It's hard to say how many total calories per day anyone needs to maintain his or her weight, because so many variables play into calorie requirements. Exercise is a big factor. The more physically active teens are, the more calories they need. Taller and heavier teens need more calories than shorter and lighter teens of the same age and activity level. And because muscle tissue burns more calories than fat tissue, muscular teens generally burn more calories than flabby teens of the same age and size. There's also variation from one teen to the next depending on where they are in puberty. When teens are going through a growth spurt, calorie needs increase. And adolescent boys generally need more calories than girls of the same age.

The following chart provides some sense of how many calories a healthy teen needs to maintain his or her weight. These values represent the estimated number of calories needed each day by typical (not overweight) young people at various ages.

	Age (Years)	Estimated Daily Calorie Requirements
Females	9–13	1,600–2,200
	14–18	1,800–2,400
	19–30	2,000–2,400
Males	9–13	1,800–2,600
	14–18	2,200–3,200
	19–30	2,400–3,000

SOURCE: U.S. Department of Health and Human Services and U.S. Department of Agriculture, *Dietary Guidelines for Americans*, 2005.

NOTE: These values are based on Estimated Energy Requirements from the Institute of Medicine Dietary Reference Intakes macronutrients report, 2002, and are based on median height and weight for children up to age eighteen and on median height and weight for that height to give a BMI of 21.5 for adult females and 22.5 for adult males.

For each age category in the chart, physically inactive teens would be on the low end of the calorie ranges; very active teens would be on the high end. Overweight teens in each age group who are maintaining would be expected to need a higher calorie range than the one in the table because it takes more calories to maintain a bigger body. Note that calorie needs drop somewhat after someone loses weight. For instance, if a teen maintained her former 200-pound weight on 2,800 calories a day, she won't be able to eat that much if she wants to maintain her weight at 150 pounds.

Girls have a hard time getting the nutrients they need if they eat fewer than 1,600 calories per day, according to the Web site GirlsHealth.gov (www.4girls.gov), sponsored by the U.S. Department of Health and Human Services. A number of experts I consulted felt that the minimum for boys would be about 1,800 calories. (Even at these acceptable calorie levels, it might be wise to take a multivitamin/mineral supplement.)

Another reason drastic calorie restriction is unwise is that it can slow down metabolism. Although there hasn't been research on this in children, studies in adults suggest that when someone cuts back too much on calories, the body seems to say, "You're not feeding me enough calories, so I'll slow down the rate at which I burn them." If teens cut back too much and for too long, they can feel tired and moody, lack concentration, and experience hair loss, brittle fingernails, dark circles under their eyes, and weak and shrunken muscles. Growth could even be stunted, and some of the changes associated with puberty might be delayed.

How long will it take for an overweight teen to get to a desired weight? Let's say that a sixteen-year-old girl who's 5'5" tall and weighs 175 pounds wants to get down to 140. We'll assume that she's not very active and is currently maintaining her weight while eating 2,600 calories a day. If she cuts back her calorie level to 2,100 calories per day, she'll be eating 500 calories less than she's burning. So her calorie deficit for one week would be 7 days x 500 = 3,500 calories. Since 3,500 is the approximate number of calories in a pound of body weight, she should lose about 1 pound per week on her 2,100-calorie plan—and that would add up to 12 pounds over the summer. On a 1,600-calorie plan, she'd lose 2 pounds per week. As mentioned earlier, weight loss tends to become a bit slower as the body "shrinks." The good news is that a teen can offset this by pumping up his or her activity.

About 4 out of 10 teens gave up certain foods completely—most commonly fatty items such as fried foods and sugary items such as regular soda and sweets. By contrast, 1 out of 4 teens didn't cut out anything—they ate all foods, but in smaller amounts.

The bottom line is that the vast majority of the teens lost weight the old-fashioned way—by making sensible changes in their food and exercise habits—not by going to extremes.

What Helped the Most?

Interestingly, although about half of the teens went to a program, not many of them listed that as the most helpful thing they did. Rather, they were more likely to list specific steps or strategies as their "most important things" to arrive at a healthier weight. And many of them couldn't pinpoint just one strategy—they credited several as being "most helpful." As Katie S. says, "It's hard to say one variable was most important."

Once again, at the top of the list, way ahead of all the other responses, came comments about exercise. Next came remarks about eating sensibly or more healthfully. Actually, a number of teens mentioned both exercise and eating sensibly, which goes along with studies showing that the most effective way to lose weight and keep it off is to combine physical activity and changes in eating habits.

Sandra D. says that what helped her most was that she "started to go to the gym at least three times a week and paid a lot more attention to the nutrition labels on my favorite foods and all foods." For Katie S., "it was equal—between exercising three to five days a week and watching my diet, including calories, carbs, and protein intake." Speaking of carbs, just one person listed "cutting carbs" as a most important strategy—perhaps surprising given that the teens completed their questionnaires during the peak of the low-carb diet craze.

Remarks about watching portion size tied for the number three spot with comments about dieting or following a particular diet. (How-

The Lowdown on
Low-Carb Diets

Given that I recruited teens during the height of the low-carb diet craze, I find it curious that only seven of them said that they lost weight by following such a diet. Just one of them mentioned specifically that she followed the Atkins diet, probably the most famous of the low-carb regimens. Two of the low-carb followers went to Curves, an exercise facility that offers either a "higher-protein" or a "higher-carb" diet. And Eric D. cut back on carbs because of his weight loss surgery. Several of the teens did their own thing, cutting back on carbs and increasing protein, although some who said they ate low-carb just switched to healthier eating, cutting back on sugary and junk foods.

Low-carb diets recommend cutting way back on high-carbohydrate foods such as bread, cereal, pasta, rice, sweets (including sugar), fruit, and root vegetables. In their place, the dieter eats plenty of protein-rich foods, including meat, fish, poultry, eggs, and cheese. Purporters of some versions of these diets suggest that if you restrict carbs, you can eat as much as you want of foods such as fatty meats, butter, and cheese and still lose weight.

Until recently, few studies had tested these diets to see if they work better than traditional low-calorie diets that are higher in carbs. Researchers are now putting low-carb diets to the test, and a small number of studies, involving relatively small numbers of people, have shown that low-carb dieters did, in fact, lose more weight than higher-carb dieters after six months. (In most cases, the differences were not big.) However, in two studies that lasted for one year, low-carb dieters lost more weight initially, but at the end of the year, their weight loss was essentially the same as that of dieters who ate more carbs. Thus, although low-carb diets may have an edge in the short run, there's no evidence that they are more effective than regular low-calorie diets over the long term. (A big U.S. government study is testing low-carb diets further for their efficacy and safety.)

Respected Danish researcher Arne Astrup, M.D., and his colleagues reviewed low-carb diet studies—including one involving a small number of teens who were followed for just twelve weeks—in the medical journal *Lancet*. They concluded that until more long-term studies are done, "low-carbohydrate diets cannot be recommended." They added, "Scientifically, the most solid current recommendation for people who want to lose weight and keep weight off is a permanent switch to a diet reduced in calories and fat in combination with physical activity." This is exactly the kind of food route described by most of the teens.

People who lose weight on low-carb diets do so not because of something "magical" about carbohydrate restriction, but mainly because they wind up cutting calories. (The diets are monotonous, so people eat less.) And some of the initial weight loss is water weight that's regained when people go off the diet.

Another reason low-carb diets may help some people eat less is that diets higher in protein seem to be more satisfying than lower-protein diets, and people may be less hungry on them. There's also evidence that high-protein diets may ever so slightly rev up the metabolism. But until studies are done in which people follow these diets for a long time, experts won't know if they have lasting value for weight loss or if they are safe, particularly for teens.

Dr. Astrup does not recommend high-protein, low-carb diets for young people, pointing to their lack of fruits, vegetables, and whole-grain breads and cereals. Also, on some low-carb, high-protein diets, people are likely to eat too much unhealthy saturated fat, the kind that's linked with heart disease. In addition, Dr. Astrup has questions about the safety of low-carb diets for young people and points out some unpleasant side effects reported more frequently on low-carb diets than on low-fat diets: halitosis (bad breath), muscle cramps, diarrhea, general weakness, and rashes.

In a recent Medscape article, David Katz, M.D., of Yale University writes, "What, then, is wrong with recommending carbohydrate restriction for weight loss in adolescence? Virtually everything . . . There are volumes of evidence from diverse sources telling us that diets rich in whole grains, fruits, and vegetables promote health. Such diets reduce the risk of cancer, diabetes, and cardiovascular disease. Such dietary practices are also consistently, and convincingly, associated with lasting weight control, a far more meaningful outcome than short-term weight loss."

ever, only five of these kids actually followed what would be considered a "diet.") In fourth place came credit to specific programs.

The remaining answers included comments about drinking more water, eating less fat, getting support, giving up regular soda, watching calories, eating less junk food, and snacking less. Kacey L. says the most important thing she did to lose 32 pounds was "quit drinking orange juice and apple juice, because they're high in sugar and calories. And I started taking my lunch to school." Joe M. credits both exercise and the Health Management Resources program he went to as the most effective strategies. He says, "The social support of the program was critical."

GOING IT ALONE: WES G.'S STORY

My son was a loner when it came to dealing with his weight, which crept up to 270 pounds over the course of middle school and high school. Before he found a way to slim down in his senior year in high school, Wes tried many self-concocted weight loss schemes. He says, "I was always looking for a quick fix — cutting out certain foods entirely, strictly limiting my calories and fat, or half-starving myself on certain days. I tended to dedicate myself for a day or two until I made one mistake. Then I'd feel like a failure and give up entirely."

Most of the time, I didn't even know Wes was doing these things. One scheme I do remember is what I call the "Jell-O for dessert" diet he went on in eighth grade. He cut back on everything, gave up all snacking, and replaced his gigantic nightly bowl of ice cream with diet Jell-O. He lost 20 pounds. He says, "I felt totally deprived and gained it all back — plus some."

Wes came to me from time to time looking for advice. Sometimes he wanted me to dictate exactly what he should eat. When I told him that I wouldn't be his dictator but would be happy to help him make his own decisions about how to eat less, he wanted no part of it. One time Wes decided that because I'm quite slim, he'd simply eat whatever I ate.

When I pointed out that a mainstay of my diet was vegetables and that he didn't really like anything green in color, that pretty much ruled out the "eat like Mom" diet.

Wes finally decided that he wanted to get down to 200 pounds by the time he left for college, which was about a year away. He figured out the pace he would have to set and decided to restrict his calories to 1,800 per day. Within a few weeks, however, he says he dropped that down to about 1,500 calories to speed up his weight loss. Every day, he carefully kept track of everything he ate and totaled the calories frequently throughout the day to see where he was at. He used a daily planner as his food diary, where he also recorded his weight every Monday. He says he came up with calorie counts for foods by looking at food labels, guesstimating from having grown up in a health-conscious home, and sometimes looking up foods in a giant calorie book I'd given him years earlier. He stopped losing weight 5 pounds short of his goal, but he felt comfortable at 205 and has kept those 65 pounds off to this day.

I had no idea Wes was doing these things until I started to notice he was getting slimmer. The 1,500-calorie level was too low for an adolescent boy. (Males who lose weight on their own shouldn't go below 1,800 calories per day.) But since he didn't weigh or measure foods, and since most people underestimate how much they eat, it's reasonable to assume that he was probably getting enough calories.

As an independent, headstrong kid, Wes needed to do things his way. He says, "It was very important to me that I lose weight on my own, for myself." From the time Wes was a little boy, he liked numbers and was very good at math. That's why the "numbers game" appealed to him, whereas it might bore many others. Wes adds, "The journal was a very exact scientific method for tracking my progress and food intake."

But there was much more to Wes's approach than math. "This approach worked because I couldn't lie to myself. Everything I ate was right there in writing, so the journal served as my conscience. It also helped me get over minor failures, since I could see how far I'd come. I think the best part of my approach was that it allowed me to take one day at a time while at the same time looking at the big picture. Ultimately, the motivation I got from looking at my journal helped me make the changes I'd made permanent."

This approach was a far cry from his deprivation methods of the past. For a while, he did give up his bedtime bowl of ice cream. But with time, he found that he could occasionally add that back—in a smaller amount—without gaining weight.

Although Wes had been very physically active and involved in a lot of sports as a small child, he'd become a couch potato by the time he reached middle school. That's why, he says, "I wanted to tackle my weight issue by focusing on food rather than exercise—since I had such low energy when I was heavier." But he found that as he lost weight, his energy level went up, and he subsequently started playing pickup basketball games with friends several nights a week for an hour or two. Wes says, "This gave a much-needed boost to my weight loss, and it also helped to take my mind off food, since I was used to eating out of boredom."

The hardest part, he says, was simply getting over old habits. "Sometimes I think I liked the thought of having a bowl of ice cream every night more than the ice cream itself."

Today Wes doesn't feel as if he's on any sort of diet. He no longer keeps a journal and weighs himself only about once a month. He says, "I don't even have to think about eating healthy or not eating too much anymore—it's simply my way of life."

THE LONER ROUTE

The loners used a combination of approaches to lose weight. Nineteen-year-old Kyle B., who lost 30 pounds on his own more than two years ago, exercised more and ate less. He counted calories; followed a low-fat, low-calorie diet; and eliminated certain foods altogether. He says, "I stopped eating potato chips, French fries, most other fried foods, and soda. I also drank a lot of water and kept busy so food wasn't on my mind." His most important strategy was exercise. He ran, lifted weights, and used a ski machine. Marie P., who has kept off 55 pounds for more than five years, says she lost weight by "watching how often I ate and learning as much as I could about healthy eating." She also cut back on foods high in fat and counted calories, keeping them in the 1,500-to-1,800 range. For exercise, she joined a number of high school sports teams and started working out on her own at the gym.

I was curious to see if the loners and the teens who participated in programs used different strategies to get to a healthier weight. I guessed that the loners would be more likely to say that they needed the structure of going on a diet or counting calories, but they were not. Although not many teens said they were meal skippers, the loners were more likely to have skipped meals and to have stopped eating certain foods completely. (This may reflect a lack of guidance about healthful eating when trying to lose weight, as well as eating habits that were a bit more restrictive.) However, the loners also were more likely to say that they increased their exercise when losing, as well as being more likely to cut back on foods high in fat—both healthful strategies.

The loners also tended to be older when they began to slim down. Their average age was almost sixteen and a half, while the average age for the teens who used programs was just over fourteen and a half. Perhaps younger teens and their families felt more need for guidance than did older teens.

THE SUMMER WEIGHT CAMP EXPERIENCE: SARA G.'S STORY

Before fifteen-year-old Sara G. arrived at her healthy weight of 117 (she's 5'1") with the help of a summer weight camp, she'd tried almost everything to take off weight. When she was about ten, her parents took her to a nutritionist, who would "try different healthy foods" with her, but she didn't like "being dragged to it." Sara also went on various diets: Atkins, Weight Watchers (she got the diet plan from her mother), low fat, low sugar — you name it. Nothing worked. Sara said that one time she even tried to make herself throw up to lose weight ("I hated it") and another time she fasted for two days ("I felt sick and useless").

What worked was going to Camp Pocono Trails, in Reeders, Pennsylvania. At the time, she was thirteen, weighed 144 pounds, and stood less than 5' tall. Her parents suggested the idea. Sara says, "I was scared at first because it was new and I knew there would be a lot of exercise at camp. I was such a lazy person. But it turned out that people were there who could help you, and other new kids were in the same boat."

The routine was typical of a summer camp: meals followed by a sport, arts and crafts, or aerobics; some rest time; a free-choice activity; more sports; and some enjoyable evening activities. She says that everyone — both girls and boys of all ages — got the same overall amount of food unless he or she was on maintenance, in which case the kid got more food. The food was good, with lots of choices at all meals, and there was a nice salad bar. Vegetarian options were available. "Dinner is the best meal," she says. "They have great low-fat desserts — peanut butter pie, Fudgsicles, pudding. And you can have all the diet Jell-O you want." She adds, "There are people who serve you and watch to make sure you don't take more food than you're supposed to. But there are always certain kids who sneak some extras."

Once or twice a week, campers took part in a nutrition class taught by a dietitian. For that, they might have a cooking demonstration of a healthful recipe, followed by a taste test of whatever was made. Sara says, "During nutrition class, they get you focused on when you go home." A self-esteem class was offered once a week.

On Sunday, campers individually weighed in on a scale away from the other kids in the presence of the camp owner and a nutritionist. "If you don't lose, they just tell you to stay with it," Sara says. "The owner might say, 'Up a pound.' Most kids call their parents afterward to tell them the results." A number of nutrition classes were held on parent visiting days.

Sara stayed at camp for eight weeks and lost 19 pounds. But when she went home, she regained the weight over the school year. The next summer, she returned and lost 14 pounds. This time, she kept the weight off until spring, but then she started to regain it. That's when she recognized that she needed to continue doing the things she did at camp if she was going to keep the weight off.

That summer, she went back to camp for a third time and lost more weight. Ultimately, Sara lost a total of 27 pounds and grew another two inches. Soon she'll "graduate" to become one of the camp counselors.

When I asked Sara if there was any downside to weight camp, she said, "The hardest part was getting used to all the exercise. It's rough in the beginning, but the counselors help you get involved." She adds, "Sometimes I'd still be hungry after a meal. Then I'd go to the salad bar, where you can eat as much as you want, and I'd be fine." She says that camp is expensive, but that her parents have always put aside money for their kids to go to camp each summer.

Sara notes that the transition to home can be difficult. "You're surrounded by food every day—the food court at the mall, vending machines at school. When they go home, some kids forget all they learned and did at camp. But I didn't. I was so much happier with myself that I stayed with it." She adds that during the school year, she occasionally gets a call from someone at the camp to see how she's doing, and that the camp sends out periodic newsletters.

It helps that her family is supportive and health conscious. Sara says, "My parents always give me compliments, which boosts my self-esteem." Her dad told me, "We all watch our weight and what we buy at the supermarket." Sara confirms, "My parents are healthy and always exercising." Even her brother has changed his eating habits and is now more aware of what he eats than he used to be.

Choosing a Food Route

Overall, the teens used these routes to slim down.

The eat less/eat more route. Quite a few teens — both program teens and loners — took the eat less/eat more route, cutting back on foods that have little redeeming nutritional value and eating more healthful foods. Paul H., who lost more than 50 pounds three years ago, when he was seventeen, was "a soda fanatic." He switched to diet soda. He also cut back on fatty foods and snack items, ate smaller portions in general, and started eating more fruits and salads.

Similarly, Rebecca M., who began losing 51 pounds about four years ago, when she was fifteen, says that she lost weight by cutting back on fatty foods and giving up chips, fries, regular (full-fat) salad dressing, and soda. "I gradually started to cut my portions. Then I gradually stopped eating things that were high in fat or calories. It was easier for me to slowly reduce these foods and my portions than just change everything in one day. I didn't stop eating a Sunday-morning doughnut until about a month and a half after I started my weight loss plan. Choosing not to eat that doughnut and having a banana instead was just the next step in the process." (Now she occasionally allows herself some higher-fat foods, such as Doritos chips, chicken fingers, or a meatball sandwich — but "not very often.")

This approach is consistent with advice from health care professionals who believe that restricting calories, counting calories, or prescribing diets is inappropriate for teens. It's also the safest route for teens who are trying to slim down on their own. Although it's a logical place to start, the eat less/eat more method may not be aggressive enough for teens who have a serious weight problem.

The structured route. Some of the teens did better with a specific food plan that tells how many daily servings to eat from various food groups and what portion sizes to eat — all of which should add up to a total daily calorie intake that results in weight loss at a safe rate or weight maintenance, if the goal is growing into a particular weight.

Teens who went to summer weight camps were essentially on a structured plan because meals at set calorie levels were provided. Similarly, those who went to commercial programs and were given a specific food plan followed the structured route. Linda Y., who went to the Take Off Pounds Sensibly (TOPS) program, followed a diet that was "based on exchanges, fat, and calories." An exchange diet is usually a balanced food plan consisting of lists of foods with similar nutritional value, with recommendations for how many servings from each group the person should eat each day. Some professionals are opposed to teens using structured diet plans, but such plans can be helpful if they are designed with the help of a legitimate weight loss program or health care professional (such as a registered dietitian) who has knowledge of the needs of teens.

The counting route. Twenty-nine of the teens, including my son Wes, counted calories to lose weight. Other forms of counting are keeping track of the number of grams of fat or carbohydrate in foods, but only one teen, who has diabetes, specifically mentioned counting carb grams, and two other teens said that they counted fat grams to lose weight. The counting route can be tedious and may make some teens obsessive, so it's not for everyone.

One of the reasons why professional help is recommended for teens who are trying to lose weight is that it's tricky to make sure that they are getting a well-balanced diet. Of the calorie-counting teens, quite a few said that their calorie levels were lower than the 1,600 to 1,800 minimum recommended for those losing weight on their own. However, about half of these teens were in programs or working with professionals, who should have provided guidance to ensure a nutritious diet. Of the loners who counted calories, only one reported a level low enough to concern me. Once again, people tend to underestimate how much they eat. And, according to Dale Schoeller, Ph.D., an expert on calorie needs at the University of Wisconsin–Madison, studies indicate that although both normal-weight and overweight teens and adults tend to think they've eaten fewer calories than they actually have, overweight people appear to underestimate more, perhaps by as much as 40 percent. This isn't to suggest that people are being deceptive. They're just not aware of how many calories they're actually eating.

WITH A DIETITIAN'S HELP: ALYSSA AND ASHLEY M.'S STORY

Identical twins Alyssa and Ashley M. not only look exactly alike but also have nearly identical voices. But by the end of our phone conversation, I could tell that each had dealt with her weight problem in a unique way. Their route to a healthier weight had involved an eat less/eat more approach, with coaching from an experienced registered dietitian.

Previously, their mother had told me that both girls had reached their heaviest weight just before their father passed away, when the girls were fourteen. Alyssa's highest weight was 279 and Ashley's was 250; they were both 5'4". Today, at the age of seventeen, Alyssa weighs 190 and Ashley weighs 148, and both have grown one inch.

Before they found their way to a healthier weight, the twins' mother took them to two respected hospital-based children's weight programs in Boston. "These programs didn't work," Ashley says. Looking back on it now, Mrs. M. feels that one reason is because all the instruction was done with groups of kids. "Alyssa and Ashley needed an individualized approach," she explains.

Several years ago, after their yearly checkup with their pediatrician, Alyssa and her mother were sitting on their porch, and Alyssa said, "I think I'd like to see a nutritionist." To get a referral, Mrs. M. called the girls' pediatrician, who recommended Alexis Beck, a registered dietitian in private practice. Ashley wasn't keen on going. Mrs. M. said to her, "Why don't you just go one time and see what you think. If you don't like her, you don't have to go back."

Alyssa went first and was inspired by a 5-pound weight loss the first week. More important, she connected with her counselor. She explains, "We didn't just sit there and talk about weight. We talked about school and other stuff. For example, if I was having a bad week with my friends, the nutritionist would make me aware of it. We'd talk about the situation."

After seeing her sister's success, Ashley decided to go, too. Although Ms. Beck had both twins start out by keeping a detailed journal of everything they ate, she made it clear from day one that things were going to be individualized. Ashley says, "Alexis tried hard to keep things different for each of us so we wouldn't compete. She didn't want us saying things like 'Oh, I did five more minutes than you on the treadmill.'" The "noncompetitive" message worked. Alyssa says, "Since we were both losing weight at the same time, we were able to motivate each other."

Alyssa and Ashley had their own separate appointments with Ms. Beck, who gave each personalized advice about how to make healthier substitutions for foods they were eating or made suggestions for cutting back on certain foods. In the beginning, exercise was more important for Alyssa than for her sister. Since Ashley hated to exercise, she focused on eating fewer sugary foods. At one point, toward the end of their visits, Ashley counted calories, because she was having a hard time losing weight. Alyssa never counted calories.

Alyssa kept food records for a few months, then stopped. After that, she just e-mailed Ms. Beck during the week if she had "a bad day." Ashley kept food records for about four months. After that, she kept track of what she ate only when she was having trouble losing weight.

The approach toward exercise was individualized, too. Alyssa saw a personal trainer twice a week for a few months, until she figured out what to do on her own. During her workouts, she rode an exercise bike for thirty minutes and worked out on various weightlifting machines. Despite the fact that Ashley disliked exercise, she eventually started walking without being told to. She took daily thirty- to forty-five-minute walks and often rode a stationary bike for forty-five minutes.

The twins wound up making similar changes in their eating habits. They learned to eat smaller portions and to stop eating when they were full. They also started eating more filling foods that were low in calories, such as salads. According to Alyssa, "There was no diet plan. Alexis worked from our existing habits. She might suggest that I have a cereal bar instead of a candy bar or a baked potato instead of fries. But I was never told not to eat something, and I never felt like I was on a diet." Ashley adds, "We made a big point of not depriving ourselves."

Ms. Beck often contacted the sisters by e-mail between appointments to see how they were doing. Ashley says, "She would sometimes even e-mail me when she knew I had an important event that wasn't related to my weight."

Very occasionally, the twins' mother would join them in a session with Ms. Beck. Alyssa explains, "Sometimes, if I wasn't losing, Mom might come in to work on making healthier dinners. But in general, at Alexis's suggestion, our mother stayed out of it. She would never ask us things like 'Why are you eating that?' "

Mrs. M. admits that at a cost of $195 per fifty-minute session, having Alyssa and Ashley see a nutritionist was a financial hardship. In the beginning, they went on a weekly basis, but toward the end it became every other week. Mrs. M. notes, "My health insurance only paid for a small part of the expenses. I blew through most of my savings. But it was worth every penny!" (There are less expensive ways to see a registered dietitian for individual counseling. For instance, the outpatient department of a local hospital may have more reasonable rates. And some health insurance plans are more generous than others about covering nutrition counseling.)

Alyssa admits that she'd like to lose some more weight but adds, "It doesn't bother me. I'm definitely happier than when I was heavier." Ashley says, "I have a completely different mindset about food. I know when I'm hungry and when I'm not. The experience has completely changed my life. I feel a lot better about myself."

GOING THE ADULT PROGRAM ROUTE: XAVIER L.'S STORY

When Xavier L. was fourteen, his weight jumped from 305 to 315 pounds within a two-week period. That was four years ago. Today he is

6'3" and weighs 235—a weight he attained and has maintained with the help of Weight Watchers.

Before going to Weight Watchers, Xavier tried to lose weight by using Slim-Fast products for a few weeks. He lost about 10 pounds but gained it back right after he went off the plan. Another time, as part of a health kick, he gave up processed foods and began juicing a lot of fruits and vegetables in a blender. "I wasn't doing this to lose weight, but as a side effect, I dropped about 30 pounds," he explains. "I gained that weight back within a short time."

His dramatic weight gain at age fourteen was the turning point for Xavier. "It was hard enough to be the size that I was, but to have that dramatic weight gain and not know what I did to get there was devastating. When my mom heard me crying and realized what was going on, she was sympathetic."

His mother (and just about everyone else in his family) is over-

What's in a Name?

In the United States, registered dietitian, or R.D., is the primary credential that's recognized for professionals specializing in nutrition. A registered dietitian has met rigorous standards for education and training specified by the American Dietetic Association (ADA). Although some registered dietitians call themselves nutritionists, this title can be used by people without training or experience, according to the ADA. (Some states do have standards, however.) It's safe to say that all registered dietitians can be considered nutritionists, but the reverse is not necessarily true. If you consult a nutritionist, make sure he or she has at least a bachelor's degree in nutrition from an accredited college or university and training in weight management. Some registered dietitians specialize in working with children and teens. To find a registered dietitian near you who has this expertise, call the ADA's Consumer Nutrition Information Line at (800) 366-1655 or go to www.eatright.org and click on Find a Nutrition Professional.

weight, and she suggested that the two of them go to Weight Watchers together, since she had a friend who'd been successful with the program.

"The first time I went," Xavier says, "I was excited and nervous because I didn't know what the program was. I was so wrapped up in what I was feeling that I didn't notice it was almost all women. I just wanted to take it all in—to listen to what the leader and all the participants had to say."

After a few weeks, his mother switched to a Weight Watchers program at her workplace. Xavier says, "She soon stopped going but told me she was still attending her meetings." He stuck with it, however, and still attends meetings once a week. He says, "When you're there, you know you're not the only one in the world with a weight problem."

At the beginning of each meeting, everyone weighs in. During Xavier's meetings, bookmarks are given out for every five-pound weight loss, and participants get a chance to share what has helped them. (Participants also win an award when they lose 10 percent of the total weight they're trying to lose.) Next, the leader talks about the week's topic.

When I asked Xavier if the cost of the program was a hardship, he said, "Thankfully, my mother paid my way early on in the process — as long as I was losing. But now I have a job and go when I want, which is on Mondays. To me, the cost is no issue because maintaining a healthy weight greatly reduces your risk of health problems that can cause more expense. And when you reach your goal and maintain it for six weeks, you become a lifetime member. Meetings are free then."

His particular Weight Watchers meeting typically has as many as one hundred attendees. Does the fact that he's a young male in a sea of adult women bother him? "I was a little uncomfortable at first, in a room full of adults, but it hasn't been a big issue. I get a lot of attention because I'm a young person. I like being in the minority because it sets me apart from the older people. And I feel good when my leader brags about my accomplishments to everyone. It makes me feel a little more comfortable to see other guys. But they're usually older, and they all seem to be with someone else."

While losing weight, he followed Weight Watchers' flexible Points system, whereby foods are assigned point values, and it's up to you to pick and choose how you spend your points each day. "I liked having the freedom to eat what I wanted. The catch was that I had to figure out what I really did like and want. For instance, my mom would go out and buy KFC for the family. Then I'd say to myself, 'You can have just one KFC chicken breast, or you can have a salad and a sandwich.'"

Xavier adds, "If I want a piece of cheesecake, I can have it, but I have to ask myself if I want to spend my remaining points for the day that way. As time has gone on, I've found it helpful to focus more on making healthy choices and less on figuring out how I can fit in things like desserts and chips."

As for exercise, Xavier feels that it was "very lightly stressed" in his particular group, although his leader was a good role model because she exercised regularly. "She wanted us to exercise for twenty minutes a day," he says, but he didn't do much exercise until after he had lost a fair amount of weight.

Initially, Weight Watchers helped Xavier set a goal of losing just 10 percent of his weight, or about 30 pounds. He started in September and wanted to make that goal by New Year's Day, which he did. He notes, "If I had to look at the 100 pounds I needed to lose, it would have been disheartening." He was disappointed that losing the first 30 pounds didn't make a huge difference in his appearance, but he didn't give up and kept focusing on earning his bookmarks.

Xavier says he stuck with the program because he saw results. "I lost weight, and it made me more like other kids. I'm different enough because of events in my childhood. When I was heavier, I didn't have the resources to say to myself, 'You're okay because of who you are.' I went to a small school where basketball was really important for the guys. Most of them were good at sports, had flat stomachs, and wore size 32 pants. And they talked about how many girls they met at the mall on weekends. I thought, 'What's wrong with me?' My experience at Weight Watchers brought me closer to being like my peers."

Xavier said he had a hard time figuring out what his final goal should be and how to maintain his weight once he got there. He says, "My journey took over a year, and during that time, all I was was a person losing weight. When my weight dropped below 200, I didn't know how to switch from losing weight to keeping the weight off." At that point, he feels, he was on the edge of having an eating disorder. He explains, "I was physically weak and didn't look good. I'd sometimes ask myself, 'Am I losing weight or growing today?'"

Xavier doesn't blame the program for the confusion, but he did the right thing and went to his physician to find out what his maintenance weight should be. "The doctor told me that my weight was fine between 220 and 230. I needed to hear that." Xavier's weight has crept up a bit since then, but he's okay with maintaining his weight at 235 pounds. He's in college now and has set his sights on becoming a "glorified personal trainer" with a master's degree in exercise science.

Checking Out Weight Programs for Teens:
How to Find Them and What to Ask

Pediatrics or nutrition departments of medical clinics and hospitals may be able to recommend a teen weight program. Some clinics and hospitals have their own programs, and some run national programs for kids — such as Shapedown, Trim Kids, or Way to Go Kids! — or medically supervised programs such as Health Management Resources. Teens may also be able to find a youth weight program at a local university, community center, YMCA, or YWCA. Residential programs, where teens can live for a while, tend to be expensive and reserved for those who are extremely overweight.

Adult weight programs often take teens under certain conditions, but it's not known how effective these programs are for young people or how one program compares with another, particularly for teens. Some programs, such as TOPS and Weight Watchers, offer a group approach. Others, such as Jenny Craig, offer one-on-one counseling. These programs have been developed with input from weight management professionals, but the leaders of their local units and groups are not required to have a college degree in nutrition, and their backgrounds vary greatly. (See "Weight Programs Used by the Teens" for details about these programs.)

Research psychologist T. Kristian von Almen, Ph.D., one of the founders of the Trim Kids program and one of the authors of the book *Trim Kids*, advises, "When enrolling a teen in an adult-oriented program —especially if the teen is having trouble or the program isn't working out—families should be encouraged to seek out a health professional who specializes in working with teens. The health professional can then distill what's important from the program for the specific needs of an adolescent."

What Do Teens Want in a Program?

University of Minnesota adolescent weight researchers Dianne Neumark-Sztainer, Ph.D., R.D., and Mary Story, Ph.D., R.D., asked a group of sixty-one inner-city high school teens (mostly females and just over half from ethnic minorities) what they'd want in a school-based weight program for overweight teens. This is what they said.

- **A leader who understands the difficulties faced by overweight young people** — someone who's empathetic, understanding, fun loving, energetic, and able to listen. Many of the teens went of their way to say that they would prefer a leader who was or had been overweight.
- **A supportive and accepting environment** — one in which they could learn more about nutrition and physical activity and that would help them feel better about themselves and allow for discussion of personal issues not related to food or weight.
- **Fun stuff, not just classroom work.** For instance, for physical activity, their ideas included biking, playing softball or Frisbee, taking Jazzercise classes, and dancing to fast music. For nutrition-related activities, the teens wanted to do things such as cooking and eating together, buying food, and learning how to prepare healthful food.

The authors of the study said, "By far, the most commonly expressed desire was weight control. Two thirds of youth indicated they would like to lose weight; learn to maintain their loss; and/or avoid weight gain in the future."

Here are questions parents and teens may want to ask when checking out a weight program.

What is the program's overall philosophy? Make sure the program is not overly restrictive or punitive in any way and that it will enhance self-esteem. Is the approach a positive one that emphasizes lifestyle changes, not temporary fixes? According to Leonard Epstein, Ph.D., and colleagues from the State University of New York at Buffalo, the research group that conducted the most respected child obesity treatment studies available, interventions that minimize feelings of deprivation are more likely to result in lasting behavior changes than restrictive approaches. Of the teens I surveyed, Wes G., Alyssa and Ashley M., and Xavier L. all emphasized that not depriving themselves was crucial.

Does the program use a group format, an individualized approach, or both? Some teens do better with a group of peers who are in the same boat, as was the case with Xavier L. and Sara G., while others do better in a one-on-one situation, as with Ashley and Alyssa M. Working one-on-one with a professional allows suggestions for diet, exercise, and habit changes to be more personalized. Richie C. lost weight with the help of a physician who used the Shapedown program, which is designed to be a group approach, one-on-one with Richie and his family. Richie's mother told me, "He wouldn't have gone to a group. He would have clammed up."

A group approach can provide support for a teen who doesn't get a lot of help at home. Xavier says, "I sometimes feel more alone in my family of overweight people than I do when I'm with a group who are trying to do something about their weight." Groups also tend to be more cost-effective to run, so they may cost less than individualized approaches.

How does the program measure participants' progress? For instance, is a weight goal established? If so, how? Is a health care professional involved? The approach should not be overly focused on the scale, and its goals for weight loss, exercise, and behavior change should be realistic. Weighing, if done at all, should be private and handled in a positive way. At the Way to Go Kids! program that Sid J. attended with his mother, a weight loss goal is not established. Rather, the goal is to stop gaining weight and to change one's eating habits. Sid's mother told me, "The kids were weighed behind a screen. The number was never called out. The dietitian would just ask the kids if they wanted to see it." Sid adds, "If I gained a pound, she [the dietitian] never said a word."

The program should measure progress in ways other than weight loss. Changes in eating habits (such as eating more fruits and vegetables), physical activity, and fitness, as well as improvements in body composition (becoming more muscular, for instance) and medical conditions caused by being overweight, also should count. Shanisha B.'s Fit-Matters program in Chicago tracks positive changes in blood pressure and how clothing fits, as well as the ability to walk farther, faster, and with less fatigue.

What kind of food approach does the program use? Find out whether the food approach is structured or unstructured and whether different options are available if a change is needed. Teens need an eating plan that's simple, easy to follow, and well-balanced. The food plan should meet the nutritional needs of a still-growing or stopped-growing teen and accommodate cultural preferences. And unless the program is supervised medically, the food plan should not rule out specific foods or food groups. The plan should not leave a teen feeling frequent hunger pangs and should provide education about choosing appropriate portion sizes, reading labels, and eating more healthfully in both fast-food and sit-down restaurants.

Are the program's recommendations tailored to the individual? Just as one size does not fit all when trying to find a way to reach a healthier weight, one size doesn't fit all in any one particular weight program. For instance, if the program sets a suggested calorie limit, calorie suggestions should be based on the individual teen's needs. The same goes for exercise.

What ages does the program serve? If it's a program primarily for adults, do the leaders modify their approach for teenagers? If it's a children's program, do they offer a separate approach or group for teens? What works for overweight younger children doesn't necessarily work for adolescents. According to University of Michigan psychologist Jacquelynne Eccles, Ph.D., an expert on designing age-appropriate programs for youth, "Teens need to be more involved in decision making and are more likely to stick with it if they have a voice in how a program is run."

Does the program include behavior modification approaches — that is, does it provide counseling on how to change eating, activity, and personal habits? If so, how much time is devoted to this, and what types of strategies are used? Behavior modification is a catchall term for habit-changing strategies, focusing not just on eating and exercising but also on changing the circumstances and situations that lead to overeating and influence physical activity. This may involve keeping a food and exercise diary, as detailed in chapter 7.

Xavier L. says, "Weight Watchers has steps to help you visualize food situations and how you're going to react in them. They encourage you to set small goals that you can reach. They also encourage you to get rid of problem foods in your house."

What is the program's approach for increasing physical activity? Finding ways to become more physically active should not be a secondary part of the program. Ideally, the focus should be on increasing exercise and decreasing sedentary pursuits (less TV, video game, and computer time), as well as finding more ways to increase activity in a teen's daily routine (such as by taking stairs instead of escalators). The plan for increasing activity should be individualized, realistic, and based on the teen's current activity level. Shanisha B.'s program, FitMatters, included a twelve-week exercise program run by a physical therapist. Shanisha also was encouraged to wear a step counter to make sure she took at least ten thousand steps a day. She says, "I walk every day for one to two hours, and one day a week, I run for twenty minutes."

She also goes with her grandmother to work out at a low-cost gym.

How often are meetings or sessions held, and how long does the program last? It appears that when programs last longer and people stick with them, weight management is more likely to be successful. Look for a program that meets weekly for at least a couple of months, then less frequently but regularly for at least six to twelve months. Alyssa and Ashley M., for example, went to their dietitian for about two years, and Xavier L. continues to go to Weight Watchers.

Does the program have a separate maintenance component at the end? Follow-up is a useful component to help teens continue to be successful and to maintain progress. Ask if follow-up is available and if there's an extra charge for this. Richie C.'s mother stressed the importance of sticking with the maintenance part of the Shapedown program after her son slimmed down. She says, "It's as if a person has been on crutches. You want to get off them, but you can't get off them too soon, or you'll damage all the work you've done."

Does the program involve parents in meetings or sessions? Studies are unclear about how parents can best be involved in weight programs for teens. While research suggests that having parents attend sessions with the child is beneficial for younger children, it's not clear whether this works well for teens. Some programs, like FitMatters, have parents and teens meet in separate groups. Others have parents and teens meet together all the time or just some of the time. My guess is that the helpfulness of parent involvement depends on the age of the teen and the individual teen's personality, level of independence, and relationship with his or her parents. Younger teens may need more assistance in following a program. Richie C., who was just twelve when he began his program, says, "My mother came to my meetings. At home, the whole family got involved." Older teens may resist help and desire greater independence. Look for a program that suits the teen's individual preferences.

What are the credentials of the people who designed the program

and of those who have the most interaction with participants? It's best if the people in question have degrees and specialized training in the area of weight management—ideally, with young people. Find out if any physicians, mental health professionals, exercise physiologists or physical therapists, and/or registered dietitians are involved. If the caregivers are not health care professionals, is medical supervision recommended, as it should be for teens?

Can the program provide any data on how teens do in the program? Ask how many pounds, on average, participants in the program have lost. Stanford University's Thomas Robinson, M.D., says that he would ask about indications that the program is meeting participants' needs, as measured by things such as attendance rates, ability to retain participants for the entire length of the program (or the opposite, dropout rates), and satisfaction ratings from participants. Can the leaders give you names of any people who have taken part in the program and might be willing to talk with you? And do they have any information on how teens fare after leaving the program?

What's the total cost of the program? And are there fees or costs for additional items, such as food or supplements? Costs vary greatly. Sometimes health insurance will cover some of the expenses, particularly if a teen has a medical problem related to weight and a physician has made a referral. But in a 2004 issue of *Pediatrics,* Sarah Barlow, M.D., of the St. Louis University School of Medicine, writes, "Insurance companies have reimbursed poorly or not at all for pediatric weight management programs."

Be aware that in some cases, expenses for weight loss treatment are tax-deductible. And sometimes parents can save money on taxes by putting aside pretax dollars for medical expenses in health savings accounts or flexible spending accounts. A tax adviser and perhaps your employer can help you find out if your family qualifies for any of these options when paying for weight loss treatment.

QUESTIONABLE STRATEGIES

A small number of the teens I surveyed used nonideal strategies to lose weight.

Skipping meals or fasting. Fourteen teens said that they used skipping meals as a strategy when they were trying to lose weight; most skipped breakfast. A few said that they tried fasting, but none of them did it with any frequency. When one of these teens tried fasting, she says, "it made me feel sick and useless."

Using over-the-counter weight loss supplements. Three of the teens who said they used diet pills used over-the-counter supplements — either a fiber supplement, an herbal supplement, or a supplement containing a mixture of herbs and amino acids. Alison Hoppin, M.D., associate director for pediatric programs at the Massachusetts General Hospital Weight Center in Boston, addressed the use of supplements in a Medscape article on child and adolescent obesity. She wrote, "There are no well-designed studies supporting the use of dietary supplements for weight loss in children, and no supplements for weight loss can be recommended or even considered with caution."

Smoking cigarettes. Just one teen said that she smoked cigarettes to control her weight. A 2005 study in the *International Journal of Obesity* showed that sixteen- to twenty-four-year-olds who smoked were not thinner than nonsmokers. This study also showed that in women, smoking was associated with getting fatter around the waist.

Every two years, the U.S. government conducts a large survey, called the Youth Risk Behavior Survey (YRBS), of thousands of ninth through twelfth graders. In this survey, teens are asked whether they've engaged in certain unhealthy weight control activities — such as taking diet pills without a doctor's advice or making themselves vomit — during the thirty days preceding the survey. The most recent findings showed that although close to 60 percent of girls and 30 percent of boys said they were trying to lose weight, the vast majority of high schoolers did not report using any of these extreme approaches.

GETTING AGGRESSIVE:
INTENSIVE APPROACHES FOR LOSING WEIGHT

Sometimes young people who are severely overweight or have serious medical problems caused by their weight need to use intensive approaches to arrive at a healthier weight. A small number of the teens I surveyed used such approaches, all of which should be under the supervision of a physician and other health care professionals who have weight management expertise and, ideally, experience working with teens.

Meal Replacements

Five teens lost weight by using what's known as a meal replacement approach, in which you use special drinks or bars in place of some meals. Two of them used Slim-Fast products this way—one did so under her physician's supervision, and the other checked with her doctor but was advised against using this method of weight loss. Karen D., who was supervised by her doctor, used Slim-Fast to lose her first 20 pounds, then switched to Weight Watchers to lose another 100-plus pounds. (Slim-Fast recommends that those under eighteen see a doctor before following its diet.) Another teen consumed a soy-based shake or bar for breakfast and lunch. A small number of other teens used drinks and bars in place of some meals, but such use seemed to be more sporadic.

Two teens used meal replacements as part of the medically supervised weight management program Health Management Resources (HMR). Matt A. went this route because he was very overweight—280 pounds at his heaviest and just 5'7" tall—and because he was impressed with the success of an adult friend who'd lost a lot of weight with the help of HMR. Nearly two years later, Matt stands 6' tall and weighs 220 pounds. He still goes to the program. Joe M., a 6' sixteen-year-old who weighed 270 pounds, also used meal replacements as part of the HMR program. Having kept off his weight for more than a decade, he now weighs 210 pounds, stands 6'5" tall, and is twenty-seven years old.

Although it's certainly healthier to have a nutritious drink or bar than to skip meals entirely, meal replacement approaches are not advised for teens who are trying to lose weight on their own. However, James Anderson, M.D., a prominent obesity researcher from the University of Kentucky, has treated more than 150 teenagers using a low-calorie diet of several liquid meals per day along with generous servings of fruits and vegetables. He says that this approach can be effective for weight loss in teens when it's used as part of a comprehensive, medically supervised weight management program involving trained educators, lots of physical activity, and support from parents. He uses this approach only with very overweight teens who are past the peak adolescent growth spurt as determined by a physician.

Dr. Anderson believes that such programs should be used before very obese teens resort to weight loss surgery. It is unknown how effective this approach is for keeping weight off, particularly in teens. Although none of the young people in his studies have experienced eating disorders, Dr. Anderson feels that teens who are considering this or other intensive treatment for weight problems should be screened to assess whether they have such disorders or other psychiatric problems.

Medications for Weight Loss

Three of the teens, two of them sisters, reported that they were part of a study involving the use of the prescription appetite suppressant sibutramine, commercially known as Meridia. Of the two, Mia R., fifteen and a half, and Dahiana R., seventeen and a half, only Dahiana was actually on the drug. Mia got the placebo, a fact she learned when I had her ask the program she attended about the treatment. She says, "The whole time, I thought I was on the drug." Both sisters lost weight. About two years after the study ended, Mia was maintaining a 65-pound loss, while Dahiana was keeping off 80 pounds, although she had stopped taking the drug. (Mia was taller and less overweight to begin with.) Both young women also received instruction from a dietitian about how to eat more healthfully and were encouraged to exercise.

James G. took sibutramine as part of a comprehensive, medically supervised weight management program for teens. He no longer takes the drug but has kept off the 90 pounds that he lost more than two years ago.

Sibutramine, which works by increasing the levels of certain brain chemicals that help reduce appetite, is approved for use in adults by the U.S. Food and Drug Administration (FDA), but it is not approved for young people under the age of sixteen. Physicians can, however, prescribe the medication to a young person if they deem that it is in the child's best interest or if the child is taking part in a study. Other prescription appetite suppressants approved for use in adults for short periods of time are not recommended for teens.

One well-designed study involving teens, conducted by University of Pennsylvania researcher Robert Berkowitz, M.D., and colleagues, found that sibutramine had a significant weight loss advantage over a placebo for obese teens who took part in an intensive behavior modification program that emphasized making dietary changes, walking, and keeping eating and activity journals, in conjunction with parental involvement. However, the drug had to be discontinued or the dose lowered in more than 4 out of 10 study participants because it raised their blood pressure. The researchers concluded that until more is known about safety and efficacy, weight loss medications should be used only on an experimental basis with adolescents and children.

The only weight loss drug that's approved by the FDA for use in young people age twelve or older is orlistat (Xenical). None of the teens I interviewed used the drug, which works by blocking the body's absorption of dietary fat, causing it to be excreted in bowel movements. The drug's notorious side effects include oily bowel movements and possible spotting in underpants. A recent report published in the *Journal of the*

American Medical Association showed that orlistat had an advantage over a placebo in a large study involving teens who were taking part in a comprehensive, medically supervised weight management program.

Contrary to the experiences of Dahiana R. and James G., studies show that these drugs generally do not lead to dramatic weight loss. Any weight loss that does occur tends to level off after about six months of taking the drugs. When people go off the drugs, they tend to gain the weight back. It is not known how safe or effective the drugs are if used for a long time, particularly in young people.

In summary, studies supporting the use of medications for weight loss in teens are limited. These drugs should be prescribed only to seriously obese teens who have not had success with diet and exercise alone — and then only as part of a comprehensive weight management program under the guidance of a doctor or a team of experts specializing in the treatment of child and adolescent obesity.

Very Low-Calorie Diets

None of the teens in this book was on a very low-calorie diet (VLCD), sometimes used for obese children and teens under strict medical supervision. Typically, such diets provide 600 to 900 calories per day, mainly from carefully calculated amounts of high-quality protein foods such as lean meat, poultry, or fish, along with several cups of low-carbohydrate vegetables. Vitamin and mineral supplements are prescribed, along with plenty of water. The goal is to maximize body fat loss without losing body protein from organs and muscles. VLCDs are typically used for short periods of time with teens, usually four to twelve weeks.

There's some evidence that these strict diets do not have an advantage over diets that are less restrictive. In fact, Dr. James Anderson, who has conducted research on VLCDs in adults, feels that there is no advantage to having teens on such diets. "I think teens who need an intensive approach do as well when eating 1,000 to 1,200 calories per day, and I no longer use diets that are lower in calories than this," he says.

Weight Loss Surgery

Two teens underwent surgery to lose weight, called bariatric surgery. Veronica S., who had type 2 diabetes and a hiatal hernia, had surgery two years ago at Virginia Commonwealth University Medical Center in Richmond after hitting her highest weight of 330 pounds. She told me, "I was going to the doctor every other week, and I was ready to give up." Now she's down to 153 pounds (she's 5'7"), the hernia is gone, and she controls her diabetes by eating healthy foods, not with medication.

Eric D. also suffered from medical problems. He says, "I was constantly in muscle pain and out of breath from my obesity. At night, when trying to sleep, I felt like I was suffocating." He had bariatric surgery at Cincinnati Children's Hospital Medical Center when he was seventeen, weighed 385 pounds, and was 5'8" tall. Now, about a year and a half later, Eric weighs 185 pounds, which was his goal, and is two inches taller. He says, "When I walk into a room, heads turn — not because I'm obese, but because I look good and have more self-confidence. They're not distracted by my weight anymore." As a theater arts major in college, he's gone from playing the "funny fat guy, who's in the background" to playing the leading man.

Both Veronica and Eric had the most common type of obesity surgery, called the Roux-en-Y gastric bypass. This involves sectioning off part of the stomach to create a much smaller pouch, so the stomach gets full faster, and bypassing part of the small intestine, so the body can't absorb some of the calories eaten. In a consensus article on bariatric surgery for severely overweight teens published in the medical journal *Pediatrics,* this type of surgery was seen by a group of physicians who specialize in treating overweight children as the most appropriate surgical option for adolescents.

The experts who wrote the article also acknowledged another type of bariatric surgery for teens, known as adjustable gastric banding, or AGB. In this procedure, a silicone band is placed around the upper part of the stomach to create a small pouch that fills up after only a small amount of food is eaten. In the United States, a device called the Lap-

Band is the only AGB device currently available. At this writing, AGB has not been approved by the FDA for use in patients younger than eighteen, but some physicians feel that this procedure is better for teens than gastric bypass because it's less risky and it's reversible. Although initially the rate of weight loss is less dramatic, according to W. Scott Helton, M.D., chief of surgery at the University of Illinois at Chicago, "worldwide studies demonstrate that when AGB surgery is done by experienced surgeons and followed closely afterward by a comprehensive program, adults lose about the same amount of weight as those who have gastric bypass by four years [after surgery]." The University of Illinois at Chicago is one of a few medical facilities currently studying the effectiveness of AGB surgery in teens.

Weight loss surgery in teens is serious and controversial, not only because it costs a lot of money—easily upwards of $25,000, which may be covered by insurance, at least in part—but also because serious medical complications can occur. A small number of people even die as a result of the surgery. That's why it's essential that bariatric surgery for teens be performed only at medical centers with a team of experts who specialize in meeting the unique needs of overweight teens. To be considered experienced, a surgeon who performs bariatric surgery should have done at least 100 to 150 operations.

Even in experienced hands, serious medical complications can occur following the surgery, as happened in Eric's case. He explains, "My stomach accidentally became punctured during the bypass procedure, and it had to be repaired the next day. I was in the hospital much longer than anticipated—two and a half weeks instead of the several days I had originally anticipated." Veronica has had some problems, too. Several years after having the surgery, she had painful gallbladder attacks, which her physician believed were related to the operation, and she had to have her gallbladder removed.

The panel of experts who wrote the consensus article on bariatric surgery for *Pediatrics* suggests that to be eligible for bariatric surgery, a teen should have tried organized weight loss approaches for at least six months and failed; have a BMI of at least 40 with serious obesity-related medical problems or have a BMI of at least 50 with less serious problems; have finished or almost finished growing; have made a commitment to comprehensive medical and psychological evaluations before and after surgery; have a supportive family environment; be highly motivated and capable of understanding the necessary lifestyle changes, as well as the risks, side effects, and need for lifelong medical supervision; and agree to avoid becoming pregnant for at least a year after the surgery.

If they want to be successful, those who have bariatric surgery will have to adjust to eating *much* smaller amounts of food. Eric recalls, "I could eat no bites bigger than the size of a pea for the first two months to prevent clogging the opening for my 'new' stomach." According to Thomas Inge, M.D., Ph.D., an expert on adolescent gastric bypass surgery at Cincinnati Children's Hospital Medical Center, typical intake is just 500 to 800 calories per day during the first year after the surgery. Drinking three to four quarts of fluid per day is necessary to avoid dehydration. Sugary soda and most desserts must be avoided altogether, and nutrition supplements are needed for the rest of the teen's life.

Bariatric surgery does not negate the need to make permanent changes in eating and exercise patterns. Eric says, "The fear of gaining the weight back is always there. Surgery has given me a tool to help, but if I don't do the right things, I'll gain the weight back."

MAKING THE TRANSITION FROM LOSING WEIGHT TO KEEPING IT OFF

The transition from losing to maintaining can be frightening for a teen who's worked hard at slimming down and needs to figure out how to stay at his or her new weight. For teens who have been following a more restrictive approach, the transition can be even more difficult than for those who used an eat less/eat more approach. I asked the teens how they negotiated the transition from losing weight to keeping it off.

Some worked with a registered dietitian. Jon S. says, "I got to a weight that was healthy and tried to adjust my lifestyle so my eating and exercise habits maintained my new weight. But it seemed that I kept losing weight. Eventually, I met with a dietitian to make sure I was able to find that [calorie] level to maintain while in my new lifestyle."

Some went by trial and error and used the scale as a guide. Wes G. says, "It was trial and error. I paid attention to what I was eating and weighed myself once a week. If I was up a little, I'd cut back. At that point, I was familiar enough with the foods I was eating to know where I was getting too many calories."

Some used the same strategies that they used to lose weight but ate a little more. Ally S. explains, "I started adding a little back to every meal. For example, I used to only have one serving of cereal with milk for breakfast. Now I have two servings of cereal and milk. Instead of just a yogurt and salad for lunch, I'll now have yogurt, salad, and carrots with peanut butter."

Some learned more about the nutritional value of foods. To figure out what she could eat to maintain her slimmer weight, Margaret G. educated herself through magazines and books. However, she says, "I think I might have taken it a bit far with learning things that were too specific, such as calorie counts and specific vitamins. I definitely don't follow that now, but I'm aware of what I eat. I'm able to make healthier choices without over-obsessing on what I'm consuming."

Some took advantage of exercise. Stina B. had on her list of transition strategies, "And, of course, exercise, exercise, exercise!"

Some tuned in to their bodies. Amber M. emphasizes, "Being able to recognize biological hunger from psychological hunger is very important." She says it took her a long time to make the distinction. Aaron T. says of his transition, "I think that part of what happened was a reformation in the way I think about food. Now my body just knows what to eat and how much."

5
Getting Moving
— and Having a Good Time

> For me, exercise was an absolute necessity if I wanted to
> shed the pounds. I told myself it wasn't going to happen if
> I didn't exercise, and so I did. Working out can actually be
> fun if there's good music!   — Buffy S.

The teens I interviewed make it clear that becoming more physically active is critical to getting extra weight off and continues to be essential for maintaining what they've accomplished. Although some of the teens took part in organized sports, most didn't become star athletes or marathon runners. From belly-dancing to in-line skating, they figured out how to turn moving their bodies into having a good time and to reap the many benefits of physical activity.

MIKAL T.'S STORY

Mikal T. first contacted me by e-mail after she heard me speak on a public radio show when I was recruiting Native American teens — a population at particularly high risk for health problems related to being overweight — to say to others, "I took charge of my health and weight — you can do it, too!" Mikal certainly fit the bill.

A member of the Eastern Cherokees, Mikal weighed 170 pounds at her heaviest, when she was twelve. She now weighs 140 pounds and has dropped three clothing sizes. (She's now thirteen and a half and 5'9".) Mikal arrived at her new weight mainly by becoming more physically active — she joined the basketball team at her school — but she changed her eating habits as well.

Mikal began developing a weight problem at age eleven. When she was younger, she'd go running with her mother, who, in her mom's words, "had become severely overweight" after having four children. (Her mother has since lost the excess weight and is keeping it off.) When Mikal's mother started graduate school, life became more hectic, and she and Mikal had little time to run together. Before long, Mikal's weight climbed to 170. She explains, "I was a bread eater, drank too much soda pop, ate a lot of sweets, spent too much time in front of the TV, and didn't get enough exercise. Eating made me feel happy."

The consequences didn't make her happy, however. "People would make fun of me because of my height and weight," she says. The teasing became Mikal's main incentive for slimming down. "I wanted to show that I could do something instead of just eating. I learned to play basketball. Also, my grandparents had diabetes, and I didn't want to become a diabetic."

Mikal's parents were concerned about her weight, too, mainly because of the family history of diabetes. At one point, they tried putting Mikal on a low-calorie diet, but that didn't work. They'd already learned from their experience of trying to push her older brother to play football that coercing her to play a particular sport wouldn't work either. Her mother says, "We didn't want to focus on weight and appearance. So we went at it from the angle that the whole family needs to eat healthy and that all of our kids needed to be more active after school." They let their children choose their own afterschool activities, and that's when Mikal set her sights on playing basketball.

She says, "I saw how much fun it looked on TV. I also started to read sports books that said the adrenaline rush felt so good and that's why people kept playing." Reading books about sports took the place of some of her TV watching and playing video games, which she started to find boring.

Soon she went from watching and reading about sports to activity. On her own, she started doing sit-ups and pushups to get in better shape. Because she "hated the feeling of being slow, tired, out of breath, and hurting" in gym class, she also asked her physical education teacher for some tips on keeping up with the class. After Mikal expressed an interest in playing basketball, her older sister and mother worked with her on skills such as dribbling the ball. When Mikal had friends over, her mom would encourage them to go outside and do things like play basketball at a neighborhood park. Mikal adds, "My dad encouraged me to get better at basketball, but he didn't pressure me."

Before long, Mikal suggested to several of her friends (who were not overweight) that they try out for the seventh-grade basketball team with her. She made it, played well, and decided to try out for the track team next, surprising herself by running an eight-minute mile. Mikal found that she loved being active and lost 30 pounds.

While she was losing weight, Mikal says, she ate almost all foods, just less of them. In particular, she cut back on candy, and she switched from regular soda to water. For some time, her mother had already been making changes in the food department. She told me, "I try not to buy processed food, and we use low-fat mayonnaise and salad dressings. We don't have regular soda in the house. If I buy beverages, they're sugar-free, like Crystal Light. I avoid serving fried and fatty food, and much of my cooking is on the grill or in a Crock-Pot. We always have a bowl of fruit sitting around." Having family meals almost every night is a priority, too, but Mikal's mother has discovered that it's best to "make just enough for one meal," because when she makes more food, everyone eats more. For the same reason, when the family goes out to eat, they avoid buffets.

Currently, Mikal is not on a sports team, but she remains very active. Her morning walk to school is about a mile, and she participates in the marching band, which practices before and after school. Two days a week, she takes a belly-dancing class at the local YMCA. She also does belly-dancing at home and with friends when they're just goofing around.

For fun, two evenings a week, she and her younger brother go swimming at the Y. And on weekends, Mikal and other family members sometimes play basketball at a local park. She likes to make such games "even more fun" by making up her own rules, rather than "following the same boring rules you have to follow at real games." At home, she sometimes plays the Dance Dance Revolution video game.

What has all of this done for Mikal? Her mother says, "She seems more confident about her appearance and her ability to fit in with other kids. Being Native American, we're marginalized as a population, and part of that is being seen as overweight and unhealthy. Mikal's experience shows it's possible to turn the situation around."

Moving Comes First

Many things have to fall into place for a teen to be ready to lose weight, but exercise (or becoming more physically active or getting involved in sports) was the number one response to each of the following questions I asked.

How did you lose weight when you were finally successful? Exercise helped Shanti A., an Alaskan Eskimo, lose 53 pounds when she was eighteen, and she's kept it off for more than ten years. Shanti "walked more, helped elders get firewood, and cleaned more houses."

What was the *most important* thing you did to lose weight? For Spencer R., it was "exercising frequently—having a treadmill in front of the TV."

What are the three most important things you do to *maintain* your weight loss? On Cassey H.'s list for maintaining his 80-pound weight loss is "walking to school and back." He also attributes his success to lifting weights for half an hour three times a week and riding a bike three times a week for half an hour.

"Exercise more" was also the top response to the question "What do you do if you start to gain back some weight?" And it was the teens' number one piece of advice for other young people struggling with their weight. Comments about physical activity also were a major theme of parents' responses to my questions about approaches that work for over-weight kids.

"Exercise" or "Physical Activity"?

Sari M. makes a distinction between structured exercise and physical activity: "There's a difference between exercise and activity. I never go out with the mindset of 'I'm going to exercise now.' I hated it when I did. However, I'll ride my bike to and from school or work two or three days a week—forty minutes roundtrip. And I'll walk someplace rather than ride the bus. It's a lifestyle perspective, not a conscious decision to exercise."

Indeed, some experts feel that it's unrealistic to expect overweight teens to go to the Y to lift weights or work out on machines five times a week. Rather, they think it's better to emphasize the importance of becoming more physically active—walking instead of taking the bus and pursuing recreational activities such as throwing a Frisbee, in-line skating in the neighborhood, taking family walks, or playing tag. Even so, I found that most of the teens *did* engage in structured exercise, such as jogging or lifting weights, as part of their weight management efforts.

The more than 8 out of 10 teens who said exercise was one of their *weight-loss* strategies listed a potpourri of types and amounts of activity —everything from hip-hop dancing to weightlifting. Walking and running were the most common activities. Only 14 teens mentioned team sports.

When I asked Kristy C. how she began exercising, she said, "I happened upon an exercise regimen that I really loved, which led me to learn more about healthy eating." She started out at home, doing step aerobics to a video, which led her to take classes at a gym, which eventually piqued her interest in eating more healthfully. Similarly, Matthew L.'s 55-pound weight loss began at band camp, where he did a lot of marching, when he was seventeen. He says, "I noticed small changes in myself and then started eating better. One morning, I could see a little bit of muscle, and I was proud of it. That built on itself." From there, he started to run and also did some occasional swimming.

The reality is that if a teen is really overweight, it can be difficult for him or her to lose weight and keep it off without doing structured exercise or participating in sports. In *Trim Kids,* child weight and exercise expert Melinda Sothern, Ph.D., and colleagues state, "We have discovered that just *telling* families to be more physically active is not enough. Most overweight kids need weekly structured exercise goals."

Exercise appears to play an even more important role in *keeping the weight off* for the teens. At the top of Arahsa L.'s list of the most important strategies for keeping off 55 pounds is "regular exercise." She says, "I usually run a mile a couple of times a week. And just about every day, I do at least 200 crunches." Exercise comes first for Linda Y., too, who tries to walk one to two miles a day.

Although most of the teens are avid exercisers, most don't exercise every day. Nearly two thirds of them exercise three to five times a week. About 20 percent of them exercise six or seven times a week. A small number (fewer than ten) do no structured exercise at all. However, most of those who don't do formal exercise seem to be active in their daily routines. One of them, Mia R., says, "I walk everywhere. I don't know how to drive, and we don't need cars in New York City."

The length of their workouts varies greatly. Buffy S. says, "Exercise doesn't have to be that long. Shorter but more frequent activity has always worked better for me. One long workout would make me become unmotivated by being tired and just wanting to stop." She might do three 20- to 25-minute workouts over the course of a day—in the morning, afternoon, and evening. "For each of the short workouts, I'll either jog or do a quick workout from a magazine like *Seventeen.*" (Note that three 20-minute stints burns the same number of calories as one 60-minute workout doing the same activity.)

In a recent issue of the *Journal of Pediatrics,* child obesity expert William Dietz, M.D., Ph.D., points out that there hasn't been any re-

How Many Calories for How Much Exercise?

A recent study published in *Medicine and Science in Sports and Exercise*—one of the few studies that has measured the number of calories teens burn when doing various types of physical activity—suggests that girls age fifteen and up and boys age sixteen and up probably burn about the same number of calories as adults of the same weight for any particular activity done for the same length of time. Younger teens, however, probably burn more calories than adults.

The following chart shows how many calories a 154-pound adult burns by doing different types of physical activity. A lighter person would burn fewer calories, and a heavier person would burn more calories.

Moderate Physical Activities	Approximate Calories Burned per Hour
Hiking	370
Light gardening/yard work	330
Dancing	330
Golf (walking and carrying clubs)	330
Bicycling (<10 mph)	290
Walking (3.5 mph)	280
Weightlifting (general light workout)	220
Stretching	180
Vigorous Physical Activities	
Running/jogging (5 mph)	590
Bicycling (>10 mph)	590
Swimming (slow, freestyle laps)	510
Aerobics	480
Walking, brisk (4.5 mph)	460
Heavy yard work (like chopping wood)	440
Weightlifting (vigorous effort)	440
Basketball (vigorous)	440

SOURCE: U.S. Department of Health and Human Services and U.S. Department of Agriculture, *Dietary Guidelines for Americans*, 2005.

NOTE: The calorie values listed above include calories used by the activity, as well as calories used for normal body functions. For more on calorie expenditure for various activities, go to www.mypyramidtracker.gov or www.caloriesperhour.com.

search conducted on how much activity formerly overweight teens need to maintain their weight loss. However, according to the 2005 *Dietary Guidelines for Americans*, "to sustain weight loss for previously overweight/obese people, about sixty to ninety minutes of moderate-intensity physical activity per day is recommended." (That recommendation is drawn from studies on adults.) Physical activity for young people, of course, includes things such as active playing outdoors, chores (raking, mowing, and vacuuming), walking to school, and actively participating in physical education at school.

Note that it is possible to do too much exercise, resulting in a kind of exercise obsession. The main thing is to keep an eye on whether the activity seems to be enjoyable or is more of a compulsion. Signs that teens might be carrying exercise too far include neglecting other activities (such as homework or social events) for the sake of exercise or working out when they're not feeling well.

The Many Ways the Teens Move to Keep the Weight Off

As the following chart shows, the teens are active in a variety of ways. Eight out of 10 said that they engage in more than one form of activity.

Type of Exercise	Number of Teens
Strength training/weightlifting	46
Running/jogging	40
Walking	32
Using stationary equipment (bicycles, elliptical machines, stair-climbers, etc.), cardio exercise, or exercise videos	26
Organized team sports	23
Calisthenics/stretching	13
Bicycling	11
Boxing/kickboxing or Tae Bo	7
Skating (in-line or on ice)	6
Dancing/hip-hop dancing	5

Swimming (not on a team)	4
Curves workouts	4
Aerobics/step classes	4
Pilates	3
Yoga/tai chi	3
Tennis/racquetball	2

- **Angel W.** walks for an hour one day a week and also does a thirty-minute exercise video three times a week. Twice a week, she has a thirty-minute gym class at school. She also tries to walk places instead of driving.
- **Eleck F.** takes a step aerobics class at his college gym twice a week for forty-five minutes, as well as a forty-five-minute kickboxing class twice a week. He also lifts weights three times a week for about an hour.
- **Paula D.** tries to exercise three days a week for at least thirty minutes, switching between step aerobics and swimming. She also does some hip-hop dancing, kickboxing, and yoga.
- **Jon M.** does a combination of weightlifting and cardio machines three times a week for one and a half to two hours. He also plays tennis or racquetball one or two times a week for about one and a half hours.

The Teens' Ultimate Combination

I was surprised to find that strength training is the most common single form of exercise the teens do. Twenty females and 26 males do strength training of some sort. I found, too, that almost every teen who does this also engages in some form of aerobic activity, which works the heart and lungs. Indeed, when it comes to weight control, a review of studies on the connection between exercise and child obesity published in the *British Journal of Sports Medicine* concluded that the greatest weight loss benefits were seen in studies that combined strength training with aerobic exercise, which would include activities such as brisk walking, jog-

How One Teen Became a Star Athlete

Tyler D. began gaining excess weight at the age of nine, when his doctor placed him on powerful oral steroid medications for his severe asthma. His mother says, "I was reassured by the physician that whatever weight Ty gained would come off after the medication was terminated. However, the psychological effect of the weight gain took over, and his attempts to lose weight failed. The teasing and his inability to exercise because of asthma attacks continued his downslide. Ty then became even more sedentary, and this created a cycle with more weight gain." At the age of thirteen, he weighed 185 pounds and he was 5'4" tall.

Finally, when he got to the seventh grade, Tyler got sick of being overweight and being teased and just made up his mind that he wasn't going to gain another pound. He wanted to lift weights with his older brothers at the YMCA but was told he was too young to use the equipment. He tried swimming but found he was allergic to the chlorine. He joined the middle school football team and was told he was too heavy for the position he wanted to play. Still, Ty stuck with the football team and kept his vow not to gain any more weight.

That first season, he went from 185 to 165 pounds not only because of the physical activity but also because, as he says, "when you're busy, you don't eat as much." Sometimes his asthma got in his way, but his mother says the condition pretty much corrected itself with time. He also started to form solid relationships with his fellow athletes, as he explains: "I used to think that football players were jocks, losers, and arrogant. But a lot of people make up a team, and I became friends with some of them. It became a social thing."

Later that school year, Ty, who was still carrying excess weight, went out for track, which, he notes, "is a huge step for someone who's overweight." He told me, "I wasn't going to do it, because I was the heaviest kid there." But he did try out and made the team. He wanted to run sprints, but because of his weight and inability to run fast, he wound up doing the shot put most of the time. Sometimes he did run sprints, but he was "always in the last heat." He continued to lose weight, and the next year, Ty returned to football and went back to track in the spring. He advanced slowly but surely to varsity football and became one of the front-runners on a track team that won second place in the state championship his senior year. He also received an all-state award for his athletic and academic accomplishments. Today he is a slender college student who weighs 165 pounds and is 6'1" tall.

ging, swimming laps, step aerobics, playing tennis, and bicycling.

Although it's true that muscle tissue burns more calories than fat tissue, it's not clear whether strength training makes a significant difference in how many calories people burn in a day's time. Nevertheless, strength training can help people look their best: strong muscles give a person the appearance of being more toned and fit. And although it can't "spot reduce" certain areas of the body, such as the belly or thighs, it can train muscles in specific locations, which can result in a "tighter" appearance in those spots. (Moderate strength training doesn't cause teens to "bulk up.")

Strength training can be done by using free weights, resistance bands, and/or equipment such as Cybex or Nautilus weight machines. Pushups and abdominal crunches are other forms of strength training. Experts recommend doing strength training (eight to ten different exercises) two or three days a week, with one full day of rest between workouts so the muscles have time to recover. (Or upper and lower body muscles can be worked on alternate days.) Ideally, if a teen is new to strength training, it's wise to get started with the help of a trainer who has experience with young people. The trainer should have a college degree in exercise physiology and/or certification through a national program such as the American College of Sports Medicine or National Strength and Conditioning Association.

Tyler D.'s words serve as a reminder that teens may gain a bit of weight when they first start working out, particularly doing strength training, since muscle weighs more than fat: "When I joined football and track, they had us lift weights. I found that my weight wasn't reflecting the amount of fat I had on my body, because it was being replaced with muscle. Once I realized that my weight wasn't really a reflection of my fatness anymore, I started concentrating on being a healthy person." Of course, if someone continues to burn more calories through activity than they're eating, he or she will eventually start losing weight again, offsetting the slight gain in weight from developing bigger muscles.

What About Team Sports?

Despite the high activity levels of many of the teens, most of them don't participate in team sports — only about 1 out of 5 do. Those who do, have a passion for them, however. Tyler D. says, "School-organized athletics was really my gateway into exercising. Once I knew how good it felt to be healthy, I wanted to stay healthy. High school sports are for people to get to know each other and be part of a group while being healthy at the same time."

Kacey L., who loves to play ice hockey, points to another benefit of team activities: "Sports give you a group/family setting with support and people who are all working toward the same goal."

Tyler D. says, "The worst thing you can do is not give team sports a try. If you think that all athletes are jerk jocks who will make fun of you, you're wrong. Every team has people who are there for the same reason as you. High school sports are not only for the super-popular and super-talented. Over half of my high school football team wasn't talented enough to play, but we all had a good time, and that's what high school is all about."

THE PAYBACK FROM GETTING MOVING

Getting moving can be tough for someone who's not used to it, but as the teens told me, the returns are worth it.

It gives more leeway with food. Jeana S. says, "Exercise allows me more flexibility with what I eat." Mikal T.'s mother told me that she's overheard Mikal explaining to her brothers that she gets to eat more than they do because of how active she is. And adding physical activity can speed up the process of losing weight, although it's not a magic bullet. Obviously, a half-hour walk doesn't cancel out a 1,000-calorie fast-food meal, but half-hour walks can add up if they become a regular habit.

It may help with eating less food. Jeana S. notes, "Exercise suppresses my appetite for junk." Similarly, Bella S. finds that when she's in a routine of exercising, she's better able to control portion sizes.

It eases stress and improves mood. Paula D. says, "Exercise makes me feel better and helps me keep the stress down so I do less stress eating." Sandra D. adds, "Once I started getting into the exercise routine, it became almost like meditation for me. During my workout, I started to reflect on things going on in my life and used my workout as a time to relieve any stress." Victor F. says, "Exercising allows me to maintain a cool and calm attitude." Studies suggest that physical activity does indeed decrease anxiety and depression.

It may help in school. Marie P. found that when she started working out, "not only did I feel better, but I ended up getting better grades and having more energy." In fact, some studies suggest that physical activity has a positive influence on the concentration, memory, academic performance, and classroom behavior of young people.

Getting Started

Just about anything new can make teens feel self-conscious, and starting to become physically active can be doubly tough for overweight adolescents. Tyler D. says, "It isn't an easy task getting into shape. At first everything seems so hard, you feel like giving up." Buffy S. recalls, "I'd use the gym in school, and it really bothered me when people would giggle or just even look at me while walking by. It was rough to be wearing a gym suit. But overall I got over it and started to look better the more I worked out." When Mikal T. first started playing basketball, this was an issue for her, too. She told me that she dealt with her feelings by going home, listening to some favorite music, and playing her upright bass fiddle— hitting the "dynamics" button on her amplifier. "It calmed me down," she says.

Many of the teens started out very gradually, like Matthew L., who marched in a band, then progressed to running. Proceeding slowly is especially important if a teen is out of shape or extremely overweight. As

Tyler says, "It's very easy for a person who's not used to exercising to get hurt if he or she jumps into a vigorous exercise plan too quickly. And then that might be used as an excuse not to lose weight."

A panel of experts writing in the *Journal of Pediatrics* recommended at least sixty minutes a day of moderate to vigorous activity for all school-age youth. But for teens who've been inactive, the panel advises "an incremental approach" to achieving that goal, increasing activity by 10 percent each week. Thomas McKenzie, Ph.D., an expert on child and adolescent physical activity and professor emeritus at San Diego State University, says, "To ensure that the heart and joints are in shape for vigorous physical activity, a severely overweight teen should first get clearance from a physician." (It's a good idea for any overweight teen who wants to start vigorous exercise to first get a physician's okay.) Dr. McKenzie adds that he'd rather see an overweight teen who's starting to exercise walk at a moderate pace for twenty minutes than try to run for ten. He is more concerned about injuries from exercising too hard than too long, and intense exercise is harder to stick with.

And contrary to popular opinion, the "no pain, no gain" philosophy just isn't true, particularly for young people. Dr. McKenzie says, "If a teen is doing exercise and the level is so hard that it hurts or the teen dislikes it, it's not okay." Pain or discomfort in a bone, joint, or muscle is a sign to stop exercising and consult a doctor. Exercise also should be stopped if the teen experiences any of the following: chest discomfort or pain, dizziness, severe headache, or other unusual symptoms. Such problems warrant medical attention.

6 Ways the Teens Got Moving

Here are some ways the teens got started and overcame their self-consciousness.

1. **They began at home or close to home.** Mick J. says, "When I was overweight, I was too self-conscious to exercise in public. So my mom bought a treadmill, and I was able to start exercising in the

privacy of my own home." Eleck F. got started by walking close to home—either around town or on the school's track.

2. **They exercised with other kids who were overweight.** Rose Q. joined a gym with a friend who was also trying to lose weight. She says, "It was comforting to know that we were in this together."

3. **They picked the right place.** When Sandra D. first joined a gym, she felt nervous. But after she started going on a regular basis, "the faces became familiar and the people were surprisingly friendly." Her advice to anyone planning to join a gym or health club is this: "Go where you feel most comfortable. If you're uncomfortable working out with bodybuilding men who compete over who can lift the most weight, then look for a gym more tailored to your interests, such as an all-women's gym." Currently, she goes to Curves, an exercise program designed for women.

4. **They dressed right.** Kristy C. says that she was less self-conscious when she wore clothes that gave "full coverage" rather than more revealing ones.

5. **They worked with a personal trainer.** Alyssa M. did this because her self-consciousness prevented her from following through whenever she started exercising. She says, "I'd go for about a week, but I was always embarrassed and would stop going. So I hired a personal trainer and continued working with him." Just a few sessions might be enough to get started, and sometimes places such as the YMCA have trainers who are more affordable than private ones.

6. **They realized that others admired them.** When Tyler D. first started exercising, he used to feel that people were thinking, "Oh, look at that fat kid." Now, he says, "I realize that people who are working out to be healthy—not to just impress others with their big muscles—really respect it when someone who's overweight sticks to a workout plan." He has an overweight thirteen-year-old neighbor whom he often sees in-line skating, bicycling, and running. "Every time I see her," he says, "I'm so proud of her for sticking it out. After

all, the healthiest people are not always the thinnest. It's possible to be healthy and overweight at the same time."

10 Ways the Teens Stay Moving

1. **They find the right fit.** Many teens stressed that it's critical to find something they enjoy. Elizabeth G., for instance, wasn't interested in going the team route, as her younger sisters did. For a number of years, she enjoyed taking dance lessons, but eventually her main activity became figure skating, which she's continued into college.

2. **They make it fun.** Quite a few teens make working out more enjoyable by listening to music. Katie S. says, "I always exercise with the music pumped up. It gets the adrenaline flowing and makes the time fly by."

3. **They set realistic goals and increase gradually.** Jenni O. says, "I began slowly and worked my way up. I walked a mile up and down my road. Then I started walking one way and running back the other."

4. **They make it a priority.** When I asked Tyler D. how he gets himself to stay physically active, he responded, "I keep a routine and stick to it. Once you get in the habit of exercising, you don't want to break

How One Teen Became a Runner

Aaron T. became a runner by "taking something that I was never good at when I was younger and trying to become good at it." He recalls, "In school we used to have to run a mile for fitness testing, and that was always a disaster. Running the bases in Little League, forget it—I was as slow as a snail."

When Aaron started losing his 50 pounds, he made it his goal to run a 5k race and beat his dad. Aaron says, "I worked like no other and ran and ran and used the elliptical machine." With time, he became ready for a Memorial Day weekend 5k race. "That Friday night, I went on a date with my soon-to-be first real girlfriend. Then, the next morning, I hit the road at the race and beat my dad's time. That's when I knew I was a new man."

Now, he says, "not only do I beat my dad in 5k races, but the mile that used to be a struggle in school has turned into an enjoyable five- to six-mile run when I go out. Once you've made it, there's no going back to what was. Only the present exists."

it." Likewise, Sandra D. says, "I forced myself to go to the gym regularly so it became part of my weekly routine. I started going for about an hour three times a week. And the more I went, the longer I stayed and the more often I went."

5. **They schedule it.** Ally S. marks on her calendar what days she plans to go to the gym. Kristy C. says, "If I treat my exercise time like any other class time, it reinforces my perception of exercise as important."

6. **They do it together.** A number of parents and teens emphasized that it helps when they exercise together. Kelsey W.'s mother says, "One of the things that worked when trying to help Kelsey with her weight was doing things together, like running in the park." Ally S. says, "Since my dad and I go to the same gym, we motivate each other to go." If all else fails, Margaret G. points out, "go with a dog — your own or a neighbor's."

7. **They mix it up.** Eight out of 10 teens said that they do at least two different forms of exercise. Tara G. plays soccer and softball, but she also belly-dances and does Pilates. Kristy C. says that sometimes she likes "the social aspect of being in an exercise class." But other times she likes to "zone out" and spend some time by herself, which is when she runs. Paula D. says, "I keep things fun by doing whatever exercise I feel like — whether it be a dance class, a step class, swimming, or kickboxing." There's also a health advantage to mixing up different types of activity, or doing what's called cross-training: it helps develop different muscle groups, at the same time lowering the chances of injuries caused by overusing one part of the body.

8. **They try something new.** Sixteen-year-old Rose Q. says, "Set routines get boring, so when I feel like I'm in a rut with my workouts, I'll either try out a new group class or do things outside, like go for walks and runs or go to a playground. My favorites are pull-ups on monkey bars. Going really high on the swings is a great leg workout, too."

9. **They distract themselves.** Sari M. finds that when she listens to an

audio book while working out, "it makes it easier not to concentrate on the physical activity that I'm doing."

10. **They focus on the rewards.** Instead of dwelling on the challenge of becoming more physically active, the teens focus on what they get back from it. Katie S. says, "The day that I was able to run a mile was one of the happiest days of my life." Margaret G. says, "When I get too busy to work out for a few days, I'm motivated to get back because I miss that 'feel-good' feeling." Christine F. admits, "Exercise can suck at first—you're tired, sweaty, and in some pain. Then a few weeks pass, and you see results. As soon as there were visible results, I was hooked."

Decreasing Seat Time

"Looking back," Katie S. says, "I wish my television time had been limited to two hours a day and I'd been forced to join an extracurricular activity. I may have been reluctant in the beginning, but if I found something I liked, it would have been the best thing for me."

In fact, in their advice to other parents about how to prevent weight gain in kids, quite a few of the teens' parents responded, "Limit TV, video, and computer time." Rose Q.'s mother maintains, "We have no Nintendo or PlayStation, and it's the best parenting decision we've ever made." The "official" recommendation from the U.S. Institute of Medicine and other health authorities is that the upper limit for both TV and other recreational screen time should be no more than two hours a day, which tends to be easier to implement with younger kids than older ones.

Forcing issues can backfire, though. It may work better to praise teens when they choose to be active rather than harp on them when they're sitting around. It's ideal if they come to recognize the problem themselves and deal with it their own way, as these teens did.

- **Alyssa M.** says, "Now I don't just sit in front of the TV. I generally only watch specific shows. Watching television is no longer one of my hobbies."

- **Rose Q.** sets a time limit and sticks to it to keep a handle on her TV and video game time. She says, "If you try to cut it out completely, you'll just think about it more."

- **Sandra D.** still spends a good deal of time in front of the TV, but now she's often on her elliptical trainer while watching. She says, "It's a good way for me to keep my mind off how much time I have left in my workout and helps pass the time."

- **Margaret G.** says, "I don't turn on the TV until I've gone for a walk, gone to the gym, or done some form of exercise—even if it's only ten minutes."

- **Buffy S.** recalls, "Before I lost weight, I'd come home from school and sit down right in front of the TV with a big bag of Cheetos or Doritos. When I started losing weight, I got involved in things after school, like the traveling basketball team and acting classes."

Moving Without "Exercising"

Even though most of the teens do regular, structured exercise, this isn't the only way to become more physically active. Some mentioned ways they've found to move without actually "exercising"—by becoming more active in their daily routines. Margaret G. mentioned walking to the store, work, or classes instead of driving or taking the bus (and points to the added bonus of saving on gas). Sandra D. keeps her water bottle in her upstairs refrigerator, so when she's working out in the basement, she has to go up the steps to get water. (In fact, taking stairs instead of elevators and escalators can really boost calorie expenditure if it's done regularly.) Sari M. likes to go mall walking and says, "You can look at cute clothes as an incentive and walk for hours without even knowing it."

Aaron T. boosted his desire to move more by getting one of those little step counters. At the suggestion of his nutritionist, he used it to work his way up to 10,000 steps a day.

According to *The Step Diet Book* by James Hill, Ph.D., and col-

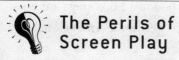

The Perils of Screen Play

A 2004 Kaiser Family Foundation report that reviewed more than forty studies on the role of media in childhood obesity concluded that the bulk of the research indicates that kids who spend more time with media are more likely to be overweight than kids who spend less time. The evidence also suggests, not surprisingly, that interventions reducing kids' media time result in weight loss.

A 2005 Kaiser Family Foundation report looked into how much recreational time a large group of third through twelfth graders spent using TV, videotapes, music, video games, computers, movies, and print media. The grand total was just under six and a half hours per day—adding up to more than a forty-hour workweek! The vast majority of this time was spent with electronic media. Of the 3 out of 4 kids who read for pleasure, average reading time was forty-three minutes per day.

Here are some other surprising findings from the report.

- Two thirds of all the kids had a TV in their bedroom, and half had a video game player there.
- More than half had a VCR or DVD player in their bedroom, and nearly a third had a computer there.
- Kids with a TV in their room spent almost ninety minutes more in a typical day watching TV than those without a set in their room.
- Those with a bedroom computer used it about forty-five minutes more per day than those who didn't.
- About half of the kids said that their parents have no rules about watching TV.
- Young people who had parent-enforced rules about watching TV reported two less hours of daily media use than those without rules.

leagues, the average number of steps a teen takes each day is 6,000 to 8,000. But this may be on the high side for overweight kids, since overweight people tend to take fewer steps than those who are not overweight. *The Step Diet Book* (which comes with a small, easy-to-use step counter) recommends that overweight teens, after determining their baseline step count, work up to at least 10,000 to 12,000 steps a day—doing it gradually, adding 500 to 1,000 steps per week. (Intentional exercise counts as part of the step count, too.)

Aaron found that activity in his daily life often helped him get close to the 10,000-step goal. But he needed intentional, structured exercise to hit and surpass the goal. He adds, "I'm not going to lie—the step counter can be a pain to wear. But no one notices, and it works well."

Two companies that offer step counters are Accusplit, (800) 935-1996, www.accusplit.com, and New-Lifestyles, (888) 748-5377, www.new-lifestyles.com.

How to Support Teens

Some of the parents stressed how important it was for them to support their teens as they became more physically active. James R.'s mother says, "Anytime James wanted to do any physical activity, we would say yes." Mikal T.'s parents continue to provide support by transporting Mikal and her brothers to and from activities, making sure they have the equipment they need, attending their games, cheering them on, and applauding their efforts regardless of how they perform. A number of parents supported their teens by paying for them to join health clubs, gyms, or summer weight camps (which tend to focus on physical activity).

Kelsey W.'s mother maintains that one of the things that helped Kelsey was buying her new sneakers and workout gear. Such support can get expensive, but there are ways to keep costs down. Mikal belongs to the YMCA. Along with community centers, such places can be less expensive than private health clubs. For a modest fee, Alyssa M. was able to use the pools, workout areas, and tennis and basketball courts at a college in her community. When Sandra D. convinced her father to buy an elliptical trainer for the family, she found one on the Internet for about $350.

Mikal's mother shares one of the best forms of support: "When

Mikal was first starting to be active, the real incentive for her was that we spent time together." Although grad school kept Mikal's mom busy and initially interfered with their runs, she made time to be active with Mikal. "We'd go running on local trails, or we'd walk to the mall instead of driving. And when we'd visit Mikal's grandparents on the reservation, we'd go for long walks together." This type of support doesn't cost a dime.

6

Eating to Keep It Off
The Teens' 10 Keys to Success

I watch the choices I make. I know I can't go back to eating
four slices of pizza and lots of junk because my weight will
bounce back. Now I eat chicken, fish, pasta, and soups —
and I like salads a lot. Water is my main beverage. I watch
my portion sizes. I know the food will be there tomorrow, or
I can take it home. I'm aware of what the reality is without
depriving myself. In fact, I still love desserts and have a
few Hershey's Kisses almost every day.   — Katie S.

Like Katie S., the teens put to work many different strategies for eating, and they avoid extremes. By using a variety of techniques, they have succeeded in staying at a weight that's right for them without an all-out "diet" effort. The strategies in this chapter also can help teens who are still overweight slim down at a slow, steady, healthy pace.

SID J.'S STORY

Sid J., who weighed 183 pounds by the time he was fourteen (he was just 5'3"), was taunted mercilessly in middle school for his weight and learning disabilities. He escaped into a world of food and movies, seeking refuge in his closetful of costumes.

Today the bright, articulate seventeen-year-old weighs 140 pounds and is four inches taller than he was at his heaviest. An aspiring film director who still loves movies, he has grown confident and now both directs and acts in high school plays. He's also gone before his local school board to advocate for other students with special needs.

Sid told me that he became overweight around the age of ten. His parents noticed it before he did. "They'd make comments like 'You shouldn't eat that fudge,'" he says. "But guilt trips didn't work on me." His mother, a nutrition-conscious nurse, now recognizes that statements like that can backfire: "Telling Sid not to eat something just didn't work, nor did nagging, bribery, or deprivation." Sid often resisted eating the healthful foods the family had on hand. Neither of his two older brothers had a weight problem, and one of them could eat a lot without gaining weight because he was an athlete.

Sid says of his eating habits at the time, "I had no limits. I ate till I got full and kept eating. When I had fast food, I'd eat all the fries that came with the order and want more. I'd eat all day and have seconds on desserts. There was no such thing as portion control." Of his parents' attempts to get him to drink Diet Coke, Sid says, "Other kids drink alcohol and do drugs. I'd sneak regular Coke, and my parents didn't know."

Sid tried some of his own schemes to lose weight, but nothing worked. Toward the end of eighth grade, his mother came to him and said she was worried about his health. She'd heard about a new kids' weight program starting at their local hospital and asked if he'd go to the first meeting to see if he liked it. Sid was receptive to the idea because his bar mitzvah was coming up and he wanted to look good.

Sid signed up for the Way to Go Kids! nutrition and fitness program developed by two registered dietitians. According to Sid's mother, who attended all the sessions, the dietitians' "accepting, encouraging, and positive approach" was evident from the first session on. His mom adds, "As a nurse, I'd given him similar information. But a dietitian isn't his mother, so he was ready to sign on." Within the first month, Sid went from 183 to 170 pounds. Sid says, "It all started working, so I kept going. I just continued doing what I learned in class, and I'm still doing it three years later."

Sid explains that the overall message of the program was moderation. He adds, "Deprivation is almost a form of torture. I feel sorry for people who say, 'I can't eat bread—oh, I shouldn't be doing this.'" In fact, one of the first things the dietitian did in the class was to have each participant put a Hershey's Kiss in his or her mouth and hold it there until she was finished talking five minutes later. The idea, Sid says, was that "it's not what you eat, but how much."

The program doesn't use a "diet" or have kids count calories, but it does emphasize making more healthful food choices. (For more on the Way to Go Kids! program, see "Weight Programs Used by the Teens.") Sid's mom says, "He'd come home from class and count out eleven Baked! Lay's chips or fifty-five Pepperidge Farm Goldfish because that's what the label lists as a portion size." He also cut back on fatty foods, such as regular hot dogs, and started eating more salads. His penchant for snacking was satisfied by healthful snacks, such as a sliced apple or banana with some peanut butter spread on the surfaces.

The program also emphasizes exercise. Sid took karate lessons and walked on the family's treadmill regularly. Currently, he does his own routine of weightlifting and calisthenics—at home, about five times a week.

Sid continues to eat a lot more salads and fruits than he did when he was heavier, but he admits that he doesn't like many green vegetables. As for soda, he says, "now, I won't drink anything *but* Diet Coke." He goes through a lot of bottled water, too, which, he says, fills him up. Instead of having seconds on chocolate cake, he eats one piece. If he "slips" and eats more than he intended, he tells himself, "Tomorrow is a new day, with a chance for a new beginning."

Like many teens, Sid has a busy schedule. For instance, play practices often keep him from eating supper with his family. His mom told me that he's always eaten breakfast—not much, but toast, cereal with milk, or a biscuit. On school days, his mother usually packs his lunch—typically a reduced-fat peanut butter and jelly sandwich on wheat bread. He continues to eat baked chips and watches the amount. In fact, he still reads labels all the time, paying particular attention to the portion size information. He eats out fairly often but is careful about what he orders. When I interviewed him, he'd just eaten at a Chili's restaurant, where he'd ordered a burger with a salad—"always with the dressing on the side and with low-fat dressing if they have it."

When I asked if any of his peers make fun of him for his food choices, he said, "It's not a problem. If someone asks me why I get Diet Coke, I just tell them I don't like the regular kind—it's too sugary. I don't owe them any other explanation." I also wondered if it's difficult for Sid to remain vigilant about his food choices. He admits, "Sometimes it is a hardship. But I remember what it was like to be fat, and I don't want to go back to that."

When I asked Sid's mother how his life has changed since he arrived at a healthier weight, she told me, "He's got friends now, and people don't make fun of him anymore. His cell phone rings all the time. He looks better, which has helped him gain more self-esteem. He's become comfortable in his own skin—he doesn't need his costumes anymore."

THE TEENS' EATING HABITS THEN AND NOW

Like Sid, virtually all of the teens described marked changes in their eating habits compared to when they were heavier. Jorgey W. and David G. sum this up well.

Jorgey W.

Then: "When I was overweight, I'd eat fast food almost every night. I'd get a double hamburger, fries, and a shake and eat all of it. At school,

---

To find out how many servings of various food groups a teen should have for a healthy diet, visit this Web site: www.pyramid.gov. For detailed information about how many servings from each food group are recommended for varying calorie levels, go to www.pyramid.gov/downloads/MyPyramid_Food_Intake_Patterns.pdf.

I'd eat my lunch and then go to the snack line and get nutty bars and/or brownies. After school, I'd pig out on chips, ice cream, cookies—basically anything I could get my hands on. Every Friday night, I used to have four slices of pepperoni pizza."

Now: After losing 120 pounds, thirteen-and-a-half-year-old Jorgey often makes her own healthy meals, such as a salad with lean meat in it. When she comes home from school, she might have a piece of fruit or an occasional cup of low-fat frozen yogurt. She says, "I was a kid who loved food, and I still do. But I took all the motivation that I had and made it so powerful that I think before I grab food. I now love healthy food!" She still has pizza a couple of times a month, but just two slices, and now it's thin-crust with veggies.

David G.

Then: "When I was at my worst, I would graze all day in the kitchen. Late at night and sometimes during the day, I would eat every snack I wanted until I was full. At meals, I would eat whatever I wanted, followed by dessert."

Now: After losing 65 pounds and growing two inches more since three years ago when he was sixteen, David keeps his weight off by eating three meals and an afternoon snack each day and by "moderating fatty and high-carb foods" such as desserts, bread, and pasta. He also gave up soda and drinks more water. When he goes out to eat, David avoids fried foods and opts for salads, soups, and other healthful choices. About once a week, he has a small dessert or special snack.

THE TEENS' 10 KEYS TO EATING SUCCESS

When I asked the teens open-ended questions about how they lost weight—and how they have kept it off—one of their most common responses was, simply, "I ate sensibly." But how did teens who'd been eating "whatever, whenever" put sensible eating into effect? They used

—and continue to use—multiple strategies, which prevent them from having to go to extremes.

Key to Success #1: They changed what they drink.

I was surprised at how often the teens made comments about changing their beverage choices. Eight out of 10 teens said they drink more water now than when they were heavier. Some, like Sid J., said it helps them to eat less. Rose Q. advises others struggling with their weight, "Drink a bottle of water before every meal. Not only does it help keep you hydrated, it fills you up a little so you don't eat as much." Aaron T. says, "A lot of the time when you feel hungry, you are just thirsty."

According to Barbara Rolls, Ph.D., a renowned expert on how to feel full on fewer calories and author of the book *The Volumetrics Eating Plan,* studies don't confirm that drinking water helps people consume fewer calories. But she suggests that it may be helpful for weight management because it substitutes for calorie-containing beverages.

Nearly two thirds (65 percent) of the teens said that they drink less regular soda. Some said that this was the most important thing they did to lose weight. Bella S. says, "I'd rather use my calories on food items instead of drinking them."

A study presented at the Experimental Biology 2005 meeting suggests that no other single food group contributes more calories to a teen's diet than soda and fruit drinks. (Fruit drinks and fruit-flavored beverages with small amounts of real fruit juice are similar to soda—little more than sugar-flavored water.)

A number of teens have switched to diet soda. A few boys said that they get razzed about this. Aaron T. has been called "a girl" for ordering Diet Coke, but, he says, "I'd rather be called a girl than be called fat." Although some people claim that diet drinks can make people gain weight, diet drinks can actually help people lose if they take the place of sugary beverages and are not used as an excuse to indulge in high-calorie solid foods. As for safety concerns about sugar substitutes such as aspartame and sucralose, reasonable amounts of these sweeteners are fine.

Many of the teens said that they now drink less juice. Although there's nothing wrong with having modest amounts of 100 percent fruit juice (without added sugar), the calories they contain can mount up. In addition, whole fruit has been shown to make people feel fuller than juice from the same fruit.

As for sports drinks, Sid J. says, "I stay away from them because, in my opinion, they're just as bad as regular soda — most of them are just sugar with some nutrients added. Unless you're a hard-core athlete, there's no need for them." He's basically right. Although the calories and nutrients in sports drinks can be helpful for athletes doing strenuous exercise for long periods of time, they can defeat at least some of the calorie-burning benefits of activity for most kids doing moderate exercise. (Check the labels to find lower-calorie sports-type drinks.)

Twenty of the teens said that they now drink more milk; 18 said that they drink less. About half said there's been little or no change in their milk drinking. As for ads suggesting that milk products help with weight loss, some studies support this, while others don't. What we can say, according to the University of British Columbia's Susan Barr, Ph.D., R.D., a researcher who has studied the connection between milk and weight, is this: "Although some teens reduce or eliminate milk products when they're trying to slim down, there is no evidence to suggest that this helps them with weight loss. In fact, weight loss diets should emphasize low-fat or nonfat milk products. Bone mass can decrease during weight loss, and this loss of bone can be reduced or possibly prevented by consuming three servings per day of milk products."

The Teens' Tips for Changing Drinks

- **Aaron T.** says, "When I was losing weight, I kept a glass of water next to me at the computer. This was the easiest way to get my water in."
- **Jeana S.** advises, "Get yourself a water bottle and carry it with you everywhere."

- **Bella S.** finds that it helps to have a glass of water before every meal.
- **McKenzie K.** says, "I often drink no-calorie flavored water, and it tastes like I'm drinking juice or pop."
- **Eric D.** says, "One of my favorite things is Crystal Light packets that you can throw in a twenty-ounce bottle of water and shake up. They taste amazing, and people just think you're drinking Kool-Aid."

Key to Success #2: They cut the fat.

Most of the teens mentioned cutting fatty foods as one of the strategies they use to maintain their weight loss. In fact, fatty foods are at the top of the list of foods they avoid. Jack F. says, "I avoid all notoriously fatty foods and greasy ways of preparing foods. I only eat fat-free salad dressing, and I never eat mayo." Sid J.'s mother recalls that his dietitian made

 Simple Substitutions, Big Savings

Any one of these simple substitutions may not seem like a big calorie savings, but they add up to a net savings of about 550 calories a day. Cutting back by that much would result in losing a bit more than a pound a week.

Substitute This	For This	Calories Saved
1 English muffin with 1 tablespoon jam	1 large blueberry muffin	197
1 oz. low-fat cheddar cheese	1 oz. regular cheddar cheese	65
3 oz. cooked extra-lean hamburger (5% fat)	3 oz. cooked regular hamburger (25% fat)	88
1 cup skim milk	1 cup whole milk	56
1 cup low-fat frozen yogurt	1 cup regular ice cream	70
3 oz. roasted chicken, skinless	3 oz. fried chicken (leg meat, w/skin)	72

NOTE: You can easily do your own searches and comparisons by going to the U.S. Department of Agriculture's National Nutrient Database at www.nal.usda.gov/fnic/foodcomp/search/index.html.

a huge impression on him when she showed the kids in the weight program test tubes with the actual amounts of fat contained in various foods. The fat in a Big Mac almost fills a test tube completely, that in a glazed doughnut fills it more than halfway, and that in a pancake barely covers the bottom of a tube.

Sid warns, however, that "something can say fat-free and still be loaded with sugar. It's not going to do you much better." He's right—some lower-fat or fat-free foods, such as reduced-fat peanut butter, have about the same number of calories as their full-fat counterparts. Watching fat and calories at the same time is most effective for managing weight.

According to the 2005 *Dietary Guidelines for Americans,* the recommended total fat intake for teens up to the age of eighteen is between 25 and 35 percent of calories. (Teens trying to manage their weight will likely find it easier to do if they stay on the low end of that range.) For older teens and adults, the recommended intake is between 20 and 35 percent of calories. For example, for someone who's maintaining his or her weight on 2,000 calories a day, 20 percent of calories from fat would be 44 grams, and 25 percent would be 56 grams. Sid J. says, "I look at the labels, and if a food has something like 30 grams of fat per portion, I'll eat less than the portion size."

Fat has more than double the calories of carbohydrate and protein on an ounce-for-ounce basis. Therefore, fat is foe to the weight-conscious because high-fat foods tend to pack more calories into a smaller volume than do low-fat foods, making it easy to consume more calories in a shorter period of time when you eat them. Excess fat calories also are more readily converted to body fat than are calories from other nutrients.

The Teens' Tips for Cutting Fat

- **They make changes gradually.** David G. says, "With time, I realized that my whole perspective had changed from 'Crap, all I can eat is this healthy stuff' to 'Geez, I'm a health nut, and I like to eat this healthy stuff.'"

- **They cut fat in half.** Sid J. says, "Just because Burger King gives you a packet of dressing doesn't mean you have to eat the whole thing."
- **They add back flavor.** Xavier L. says he uses Mrs. Dash seasoning on low-fat foods. Instead of mayo, Aaron T. "found a great mustard and stuck to it." He also uses hot sauce as a flavoring.
- **They use less fat or no fat in preparing packaged foods and recipes.** McKenzie K.'s mother says, "When we make mac and cheese mixes, we omit the butter. And when we make brownies, we use apple sauce in place of the oil."
- **They avoid fried foods.** James G. says, "When I was overweight, I'd always eat fried foods. Now I've ruled out fried foods and replace them with grilled foods — for instance, grilled fish rather than fried."
- **They use fat-free or reduced-fat dairy products.** Sid J. was amazed at how much fat he could save by using fat-free American cheese on his sandwiches in place of regular cheese — about 13 grams and close to 100 calories for two slices of cheese.
- **They use the paper-plate test.** Sandra D. offers a good tip for figuring out if prepared foods are fatty: "If the grease from the food soaks into the plate, you shouldn't eat it."
- **They cut back on fatty meat.** McKenzie K.'s mother says, "We have little to no red meat." Three teens said they're vegetarians.

Key to Success #3: They downsize portions.

Comments about downsizing portions (and eating less in general) were at the top of the list when I asked the teens, "How have your eating habits changed since you lost weight?"

Emily B. says, "Once I used portion control, I began to lose weight." A number of teens talked about the importance of reading labels when trying to decipher portion sizes. Before losing weight, Zach G. says, "I thought the nutrition facts on the label were for the whole bag or package." The first thing to look for on the label is serving size; then pay careful attention to servings per container to see how many calories, grams of fat, and other nutrients are in the amount you plan to eat.

Portion Distortion

When did 20 ounces of soda become a serving size? A 20-ounce soda has 250 calories—without the burger and fries! In the early 1980s, a 6.5-ounce soda, at 85 calories, was standard. Many of our favorite foods have been upsized in the past twenty years.

Then: A bagel was 3 inches in diameter and had 140 calories.

Now: A typical bagel is 6 inches in diameter and has 350 calories.

Then: The average cheeseburger had 333 calories.

Now: A typical fast-food cheeseburger has 590 calories.

Then: An 8-ounce cup of coffee with whole milk and sugar had 45 calories.

Now: A 16-ounce mocha coffee (with steamed whole milk and mocha syrup) has 350 calories.

Then: Movie popcorn boxes held about 5 cups of popcorn, with 270 calories.

Now: A tub of popcorn has 630 calories—and that's before the free refills.

SOURCE: The National Institutes of Health Portion Distortion Interactive Quiz and Portion Distortion II Interactive Quiz, http://hp2010.nhlbihin.netportion.

Research among adults shows quite clearly that the bigger the portion is, the more they eat. In a study by Barbara Rolls, Ph.D., and her colleagues, young men and women who were served lunch once a week for four weeks received one of four sizes of a deli-style sandwich—six, eight, ten, or twelve inches. The bigger the sandwich was, the more they ate. And several studies suggest that we don't compensate for a big meal or snack by eating less later in the day.

In another study from Dr. Rolls's lab, adults who were given four different-size portions of macaroni and cheese on different days ate 30 percent more calories when offered the largest portion compared to the smallest portion. However, they rated their degree of fullness similarly regardless of the portion size. And after the study was over, fewer than half of the participants even noticed there were differences in the portions put in front of them.

But when Dr. Rolls and her colleagues did a similar study with three-year-olds, offering them three different-size portions of mac and cheese at three separate lunches, the size of the portion didn't affect the amount they ate. Five-year-olds, however, responded like adults, eating significantly more when offered more. Somewhere along the way, it appears, something goes awry with our ability to regulate how much we eat when we are exposed to large portions. Some experts think that external influences, such as encouraging children to clean their plates, urging them to eat, and restricting certain foods, may undermine kids' internal ability to recognize their own biological signals for hunger and fullness.

The Teens' Tips for Downsizing Portions

- **They use smaller plates, cups, and bowls.** Tara G. says, "In the morning, when I go to eat cereal, I use a small bowl and fill it to the top. It makes me think I'm getting more, when, in actuality, I'm eating a normal portion size. This starts me off on the right foot and keeps me motivated to keep using portion control through the day."
- **They make less.** Aaron T. advises, "Don't cook so much food."
- **They make it a rule not to eat out of a bag or a container.** Sid J. lets the label be his guide to a single portion size.
- **They avoid serving food family style.** Molly S. says, "Don't put food in serving dishes out on the table. Instead, each person should make his own plate, with no second helpings."
- **They measure.** Nicole S. says that one of her most important strategies for maintaining her weight loss is "weighing and measuring my food." When measuring devices aren't handy, use these rough portion guides.

> 1 ounce of hard cheese = 4 dice
>
> 2 tablespoons of peanut butter = a Ping-Pong ball
>
> 1 medium potato = a computer mouse
>
> 3 ounces of meat, fish, or poultry = a deck of cards
>
> 1/2 cup of cooked rice = a cupcake wrapper full
>
> 1 cup of pasta or cereal = a fist

Key to Success #4: They eat more fruits and vegetables.
The teens fill the hunger void by eating plenty of fruits, vegetables, and salads. Sid J. says, "They fill me up, so I'm not as hungry for the fattening things." McKenzie K. says, "I go to the store with my mom and pick out lots of fruits and veggies that I like. I usually have seven servings a day of them, sometimes more." The high water content and fiber in fruits and vegetables gives them volume without a lot of calories. Studies indicate that the volume of food eaten at meals, rather than the calorie content, is what makes people feel full and stop eating.

Since fruits and vegetables do have calories, they can't be eaten in unlimited quantities, but they make good substitutes for higher-calorie ingredients. For instance, someone who's used to having a huge bowl of cereal each morning can cut the amount in half but top it off with some fruit. Or a two-inch-high deli sandwich can be spared the mayo and a couple of ounces of cheese and meat but fleshed out with added lettuce, cucumbers, onions, mushrooms, spinach, or grilled vegetables.

The Teens' Tips for Eating More Fruits and Vegetables
- **Prepare them ahead.** After going shopping with her mother to select her favorite vegetables and fruits, McKenzie K. says, "when I have some extra time, I usually wash them, cut them all up, and store them in a plastic bag. This way, if I'm on the go, it's easier to eat healthy because everything's already set to go."
- **"Experiment!"** says Xavier L. "Try something new often—like putting strawberries in a salad with light Italian dressing. It's awesome."
- **Go for color.** McKenzie K. advises, "Try eating five servings of different-colored fruits and veggies per day." Dark green and orange fruits and vegetables—such as broccoli, dark greens, carrots, winter squash, and cantaloupe—add variety plus important nutrients.
- **Add flavor.** Aaron T. says, "Sautéed spinach with garlic and a little olive oil really hits the spot."
- **"Substitute veggies for one dinner item,"** Bella S. advises. In other

words, try replacing an item that's more fattening—such as flaky dinner rolls with butter—with an extra vegetable. When looking at a dinner plate, fruits, veggies, and whole grains should take up most of the space.

- **"Eat a salad before lunch and/or dinner,"** Rose Q. suggests. In fact, studies in Dr. Barbara Rolls's lab showed that people who ate a first course of either a salad (with low-calorie dressing) or a broth-based soup (such as vegetable soup) ate fewer calories than if they had no first course.

Key to Success #5: They eat regular meals.
Leigha J. says that the number one reason she became overweight was that she ate only once a day. Now, after losing 70 pounds, she eats breakfast, lunch, and dinner, plus several snacks. Tyler D. says that he went from "eating whenever I wanted" to eating three times a day. Their new meal patterns are consistent with those of the vast majority of the teens, who said that they eat three meals a day.

Breakfast, in particular, seems to be an important meal for weight maintainers. Nearly three quarters of the teens said that they regularly eat breakfast, a morning snack, or both. This is surprising, since breakfast is the most commonly skipped meal among adolescents. In fact, one study suggested that only 29 percent of teenage girls eat breakfast daily. My finding that many teens eat in the morning is consistent with research from the National Weight Control Registry, which has surveyed thousands of adults who have lost weight and kept it off. Eight out of 10 of them said that they were daily breakfast eaters.

Twenty-year-old Tyler D., who has maintained his weight for more than six years, says, "I never used to eat anything for breakfast, but then I read a study that said eating nothing every day for breakfast is just as bad as eating a fatty piece of steak with mashed potatoes and gravy every morning. Needless to say, I eat breakfast now. Skipping meals doesn't work for me."

Although skipping breakfast isn't really tantamount to eating a fatty meal, most (but not all) studies have shown that overweight children and teens are more likely than their leaner counterparts to skip breakfast and consume a few large meals each day. It's not known if skimping on morning meals is a result of an effort to lose weight or if it actually plays a role in causing weight gain. But teen weight specialist Ann Litt, M.S., R.D., author of *The College Student's Guide to Eating Well on Campus*, has found that overweight teens who skip breakfast often wind up overeating at the end of the day.

Studies show that teens who eat breakfast tend to make more healthful food choices all day long and have diets of better all-around nutritional quality than do teens who don't eat breakfast. There's evidence, too, that eating breakfast may improve memory, test grades, and school attendance.

How can parents rally teens to eat breakfast? "Join them," Ms. Litt advises. "In my experience, teens who eat breakfast are not doing it all alone. They either eat with a parent or have a parent who is involved in fixing the meal for them."

The teens' breakfast meals aren't always traditional — either in terms of what they include or when they eat them. For instance, almonds and fruit sometimes serve as breakfast for McKenzie K. And Jorgey W. has three meals a day, but not at traditional times. She eats breakfast but skips lunch on school days. She says, "I'm usually not hungry throughout the day, and the school lunch is high in fat. So when I get home, I eat something healthy."

Nine out of 10 teens said they eat lunch. When it comes to school lunches, a number of teens brown-bag it rather than buy school fare. When Mick J. was losing weight, he started taking fruits and vegetables, bread, and cheese to school for lunch. Kristy C. suggests, "Bring sandwiches and fruit from home — or pasta. I avoid vending machines, but some offer sandwiches, soups, and granola bars. Those are good options."

Jeana S. says, "At my high school, I was one of two people who packed a lunch. When I graduated, the caption under my photo said, 'I pledge my health to crackers and tuna.' "

Some teens said that they actually eat more often now than when they were overweight. And there's evidence that eating several small meals a day, rather than one or two big ones, is good for metabolism. However, for some people, "grazing"—having small, frequent meals throughout the day—is associated with weight gain, because they tend to eat too many calories that way. The teens who said they eat more often now stressed that their portion sizes are smaller than when they were heavy. Ally S. says, "Instead of eating three large meals, I eat three moderate meals and two snacks, which satisfies my hunger throughout the day."

Fourteen teens admitted that they sometimes skip meals as part of their current weight management efforts. And 12 said they sometimes drink a liquid supplement (such as Slim-Fast) or eat an energy-type bar in place of meals. Though not ideal, that's certainly better than skipping meals altogether. None of the teens said that they fast. A few of them said that they try not to eat anything after a certain time in the evening, but it's not clear whether eating at night leads to weight gain—unless that's when overeating occurs. Total calorie intake for the day is what counts most.

Key to Success #6: They shifted their carbs.
McKenzie K. says, "Carbs are good, but too much isn't." Some teens said they've cut back on carbs in general, but many more stressed that they've curtailed their intake of high-sugar carbs by eating fewer desserts and other sweets. Amber M. avoids "simple sugars" and drinks no soda. At the same time, she favors whole-grain bread, fruits, vegetables, and beans and tries to eat plenty of fiber-rich foods. Like many of the teens, she's shifted her carbs from less healthful types to kinds that are higher in fiber, vitamins, and minerals.

Fiber Optics

- Don't be deceived by appearances. Although we tend to think that brownish grain products such as "wheat" breads are rich in fiber, you can't go by the color. Instead, check the ingredients and make sure that a whole grain is the first ingredient listed. When buying breads, cereals, and crackers, look for ingredients such as whole wheat, whole rye, whole oats, graham flour, oatmeal, bulgur, brown rice, wild rice, and whole-grain corn. Don't be deceived by terms such as multigrain, stone-ground, cracked wheat, 100 percent wheat, or seven-grain. These terms don't necessarily represent whole-grain products. Note, too, that wheat flour, enriched flour, unbleached wheat flour, and degerminated cornmeal are not whole grains.
- When selecting cereals, look for packages that say "high-fiber," a term used in the United States for products with 5 grams or more of fiber per serving. (A good source of fiber has 2.5 to 4.9 grams per serving.) To pump up fiber, add some fresh or dried fruit to cold or hot cereal.
- Don't forget that high-fiber cereal isn't just for breakfast. Either dry or with milk, it makes a great snack. Try making a trail mix with cereal, dried fruit, and a few nuts. It's good, too, as part of a yogurt parfait — layers of cereal with yogurt and fruit in a tall glass.
- To get used to high-fiber cereal, try mixing it with lower-fiber cereal favorites.
- When making muffins, waffles, pancakes, quick breads, and the like, substitute whole-wheat or oat flour for up to half of the white flour in the recipe. You may need to add a bit more leavening than the recipe calls for to compensate for this substitution.
- Try making salads with cold whole grains such as barley, bulgur, brown rice, and wild rice. Toss with low-calorie salad dressing and chopped vegetables or dried fruit.
- When serving rice or pasta, serve brown rice or whole-wheat pasta at least some of the time. To make the transition with rice, for example, start by using half white rice and half brown rice.
- Use whole grains such as barley, brown rice, and bulgur in soups and casseroles in place of refined grains such as white rice.
- Try this great sandwich idea from McKenzie K. and her family: stack slices of avocado, cucumber, pepper jack cheese, tomato, green pepper, and onion, along with lettuce, spinach, and sprouts, between two slices of whole-grain bread.

Some teens went out of their way to stress that eating more fiber has been an important weight management strategy. For instance, Aaron T. said that, with the help of a nutritionist, he ate more whole-grain foods while he was losing his 50 pounds, and he continues to do the same now.

Likewise, Jeana S. said that since losing weight, she eats more fiber-rich foods, such as fruits, vegetables, beans, and whole grains. A growing number of studies suggest that eating plenty of fiber helps with weight control — partly by helping people feel full. As with other foods, weight-conscious teens need to pay attention to portion sizes and number of servings even of healthful options in the carb category.

Key to Success #7: They don't deprive themselves.

Another strong message from the teens is that they don't deprive themselves. As Olivia C. aptly says, "It's just life. When you're a kid, you gotta let yourself stretch a little and still be a kid and eat junk food sometimes." Christine F. says, "I don't disallow foods, so I'm not tempted by forbidden things. If I crave cake, I have a piece — but not the whole cake."

When I asked the teens how often they treat themselves, more than half said they do so at least several times per month. Many said they have a treat once a week or more often. Some do so every day, but it's likely to be something modest. Marie P. says, "I allow myself one small treat per day — like a small piece of chocolate or a couple of cookies. That way, I get a little of what I'm craving without limiting myself too much." Jayden L., who used to think there were "good foods and bad foods," now has "a higher-fat, more empty-calorie snack" about once a week.

The teens offered several reasons why it is important for them to avoid deprivation.

- David G. says, "It's better if you allow small amounts of treats fairly regularly. Then you don't binge and eat a bunch of it."
- Wes G. says, "Deprivation always backfired for me. From the day I started to lose weight, it was important to me not to remove myself

completely from tempting foods and environments—not only because I occasionally wanted to eat them but also because I knew I couldn't always hide from them."

- Vincent J. says, "If I don't eat what I desire, I will keep snacking."

The Teens' Tips for Managing Cravings
The teens have evolved ways of avoiding feeling deprived, enjoying "extras," and making sure that things don't get out of hand.

- **They limit portion sizes.** Kristy C. says, "I do get cravings, and I allow myself to indulge. But I always try to keep it down to a minimum—like a piece of chocolate instead of a whole bar or bag, or small-size French fries." Katie S. advises, "If I'm craving Doritos, I buy a single-serving bag to hit the spot."
- **They have designated "extras" days.** McKenzie K. says, "On the weekends—the time I feel most tempted to eat junk—I usually have ice cream one day, or whipped cream and sprinkles."
- **They make tradeoffs.** Aaron T.'s strategy is to "think about what I eat before doing so. I can have chips with lunch if I have no cookie after dinner."
- **They enjoy "extras" in a controlled situation rather than keeping them around the house.** Jeana S. eats ice cream once a week or so, but she has it only in a restaurant or store. She says, "I don't keep it in the house."
- **They have lower-calorie versions of regular treats.** As often as once a day, Jayden L. eats 97 percent fat-free kettle corn; TCBY soft serve frozen yogurt; Skinny Cow ice cream sandwiches; or fat-free, sugar-free pudding with fat-free Cool Whip.

Key to Success #8: They snack smarter.
The teens haven't stopped snacking. More than half have an afternoon snack, and 4 out of 10 have one in the evening. But one of the major differences between how the teens eat now and how they ate when they

were heavier is that they snack smarter. Before he slimmed down, Sid J. says, his snacks were so big that "there was no between-meal snacking—there were between-meal meals!" Now his school snacks include a diet soda and a sandwich bag containing a controlled portion of Cheerios (sometimes mixed with raisins), cheese-flavored crackers, animal crackers, or Teddy Grahams. His afterschool snack might be pretzels, part of a soft pretzel, or a kiddie cup of Baskin-Robbins ice cream (sometimes regular, sometimes sugar-free).

The Teens' Tips for Snacking Smarter

- **Rose Q.** says, "Rice cakes and Light 'n Fit Smoothies are great snacks for eating on the go."
- **Marie P.** observes, "Having something with fiber and protein with every snack makes me full. If I want something sweet, I'll have peanut butter on celery or an apple. When I want something crunchy, I have baby carrots and low-fat salad dressing."
- **Sid J.** says, "I switched to a lower-fat microwave popcorn. When I order popcorn at a movie theater, I ask for an extra empty box and give half to someone else."
- **Katie S.** notes, "I eat one or two snacks a day, ranging from hummus on pita bread to yogurt to fruit to a controlled portion of kettle chips."
- **David G.** says, "I found snacks that are both tasty and healthy—rice cakes, pickles, cottage cheese, and sugar-free Jell-O, to name just a few."
- **Aaron T.** comments, "The best way for me to stop the munchies is to chew gum—the sugar-free kind, of course."

Key to Success #9: They switched restaurants.

The overwhelming majority of the teens said that their restaurant habits have changed. They now go to restaurants with healthier choices, and they've also markedly changed their ordering habits. Katie S. is typical:

"When I dine out, I pick the lighter items, like salads, fish, chicken, and some pastas."

In addition, a good number of the teens said that they eat smaller portions, and many make it a point to order fewer fatty foods. Nineteen-year-old Rebecca M., who lost 51 pounds more than four years ago, says, "This can be challenging, but I've usually been able to find something on the menu."

Seven out of 10 teens said that they have fast food no more than once a week; 27 told me that they never eat it. In contrast, a study in the *Journal of the American Dietetic Association* showed that, on average, young people ages eleven to eighteen eat at fast-food restaurants twice a week. As for dining in other types of restaurants or getting take-out, 6 out of 10 teens told me that they do so just once a week or less.

My son Wes says, "At Taco John's, I used to order one of the most fattening combo meals on the menu, and I'd dip the Potato Olés in cheese sauce. I'd finish the whole meal and still think I was hungry! When I was losing weight, I switched to having two hard-shell tacos and a small order of Potato Olés, and I stopped using the cheese sauce. And I had fast food less frequently."

Overall, fast food is short on important nutrients and long on fat and calories. A study sponsored in part by the Centers for Disease Control and Prevention found that, over time, girls who ate fast food twice a week or more gained more weight in relation to their height than did girls who ate fast food once a week or not at all.

The Teens' Tips for Eating Out

The teens have developed various strategies to take control of what they eat in restaurants.

- **They plan ahead.** Felicia S. says, "Before I go to a restaurant, I set my mind on what I'm going to eat. I fill up on water and salad and try to limit myself to one slice of bread or a roll."
- **They order smart.** At fast-food restaurants, Marie P. orders things

such as "entrée salads with low-fat protein like chicken on top, or a meal with a small hamburger, side salad, and a small fruit and yogurt parfait."

- **They get a child-size meal.** Erin D. says, "When I go to a fast-food restaurant, I'm satisfied with a kid's meal." She notes that her portion sizes are three times smaller now than when she was overweight.

- **They substitute veggies for higher-calorie extras such as fries.** Xavier L. points out, "Almost all restaurants now can give you a side of steamed vegetables instead of potatoes." Katie S. says, "I may get a chicken sandwich that comes with fries, but I'll substitute steamed veggies or a salad for the fries."

- **They box it up before they eat.** Rose Q. asks for a takeout container at the beginning of a meal so she can put half the food away before she even starts. Eric D. asks the waitperson to bring out half of his meal on a plate and to package up the other half and bring it out when he's finished eating. "This way," he says, "I never see it — out of sight, out of mind. I've only eaten half of the meal, plus I have extras for later."

- **They're choosy.** Jorgey W. looks for "little markings indicating things that are low fat." She adds, "If the menu doesn't have these, I look for stuff that's grilled, baked, broiled, or steamed. I ask the waiter to hold the butter and other fattening condiments. I get fat-free or low-fat salad dressings."

- **They check out nutrition facts.** When she was losing weight, Ally S. found it helpful to go online before going to a restaurant to see if she could find nutrition information for menu items. Numerous Web sites provide nutrition facts for various restaurants.

- **They're wary of buffets.** For Aaron T., dining hall buffets at college can be a downfall. "I take one plate, fill it up, and walk away. And I'm not afraid to waste." Some teens avoid buffets altogether.

- **They find a favorite place that works for them.** "Subway! Subway! Subway!" Katie S. says. "While I was losing weight, I ate Subway four to five times a week. I had many options, ranging from turkey to roast beef and more." Thaddeus M. says, "I eat fast food about two to three times a week, but only from Subway." Victor F. offers this tip: "At Subway, I always ask them to scoop out the bread on both sides. It definitely saves me 100-plus calories."

Key to Success #10: They party wisely.
The teens have learned to cope with a barrage of food-related events. Quite a few eat what's served in moderation, while others try to stick with healthier options. Many teens, such as Katie S., use a combination of strategies. Katie says, "Sometimes, before I go to a party, I eat something so I'll be full. Once there, I choose the lighter items. But I eat some of what I want."

The Teens' Tips for Partying Wisely
- **They scope things out and plan ahead.** Ally S. says, "I survey the food selection and plot out what I'll eat ahead of time." Some teens, like John B., "budget" what they'll eat in advance. If John's going to a party at night, he eats less during the day.
- **They focus on socializing and move away from the food.** Jeana S. says, "I stay away from the food and keep myself occupied with a low-cal drink or an activity." Ally S. eats slowly and tries to do other things, such as talk with friends, to get away from the food. Marie P. spends her time dancing.
- **They bring or provide healthy food.** When McKenzie K. hosts a gathering, she always puts out chips, candy, and a plate of veggies and dip. She says, "The veggies and dip go the fastest and seem to be the area most people gather around."
- **They splurge, then are sensible.** Aaron T., who almost never eats fast food, says, "People have to have fun sometimes. But after throwing the 'diet' out the window for the party, I make sure to be more aware of what I eat during the following days." Like other successful teens, Aaron has learned that maintaining a healthy weight doesn't mean being a food saint; it means finding the right balance.

RECOMMENDED BOOKS FOR HEALTHY EATING

Bissex, Janice Newell, and Liz Weiss. *The Moms' Guide to Meal Makeovers: Improving the Way Your Family Eats, One Meal at a Time!* New York: Broadway Books, 2004.

Fletcher, Anne M. *Eating Thin for Life: Food Secrets and Recipes from People Who Have Lost Weight and Kept It Off.* Shelburne, Vt.: Chapters, 1997.

Foco, Zonya. *Lickety-Split Meals for Health Conscious People on the Go!* Walled Lake, Mich.: ZHI Publishing, 2004.

Lichten, Joann V. *Dining Lean: How to Eat Healthy in Your Favorite Restaurants (Without Feeling Deprived).* Houston, Tex.: Nutrifit Publishing, 2000.

Litt, Ann Selkowitz. *The College Student's Guide to Eating Well on Campus.* Bethesda, Md.: Tulip Hill Press, 2005.

Ponichtera, Brenda. *Quick and Healthy Low-Fat, Carb Conscious Cooking.* The Dalles, Ore.: Scaledown Publishing, 2004.

Rolls, Barbara. *The Volumetrics Eating Plan: Techniques for Feeling Full on Fewer Calories.* New York: HarperCollins, 2005.

Shanley, Ellen, and Colleen Thompson. *Fueling the Teen Machine.* Palo Alto, Calif.: Bull Publishing, 2001.

Shield, Jodie, and Mary Catherine Mullen. *American Dietetic Association Guide to Healthy Eating for Kids: How Your Children Can Eat Smart from 5 to 12.* Hoboken, N.J.: John Wiley & Sons, 2002.

Tribole, Evelyn. *Stealth Health: How to Sneak Nutrition Painlessly into Your Diet.* New York: Viking, 1999.

U.S. Department of Health and Human Services. *A Healthier You.* Washington, D.C.: U.S. Government Printing Office, 2005. Available at http://bookstore.gpo.gov/collections/healthier_you.jsp.

Warshaw, Hope. *Eat Out, Eat Right! A Guide to Healthier Restaurant Eating,* 2nd ed. Chicago: Surrey Books, 2003.

7
Keeping Track
Developing a System of Checks and Balances

> Keeping track each day of what I ate and the minutes I exercised in a daily planner gave me a way to see my progress. It kept me motivated and helped me make sure I was honest with myself. I also liked being able to chart my success. Sometimes I still look at my old records to remember what I've done, and it reminds me of how far I've come. — **Jon M.**

The teens' experiences show that one of the most important strategies for staying on track and for monitoring progress is keeping track—not just by paying attention to what the scale says but also by doing things such as writing down what they eat. Their stories reveal that they've developed various systems of checks and balances, which can change with time.

SHANISHA B.'S STORY

By the time she was twelve, Shanisha B. was 5'7" tall and weighed 210 pounds. Her mother told me, "My daughter was born big." Shanisha says she gained weight because she didn't eat regularly and because "I wouldn't eat much during the day, then I'd eat a lot at night." She says she snacked too much (eating "five bags of chips in three minutes"), ate too many sweets and too much fast food, didn't pay attention to portion sizes, and didn't get enough exercise. Her mom adds, "I always cooked pretty healthy, but Shanisha didn't like what we ate."

As Shanisha approached the age of thirteen, she finally decided to do something about her weight. "I couldn't wear what I wanted. And I couldn't do things like run, walk, or play without resting in between." So she went to her mother and said, "Mama, I'm going into high school soon, and I want to look good." Her mother turned to Shanisha's pediatrician for advice, and they were referred to FitMatters, a comprehensive weight program at La Rabida Children's Hospital in Chicago. This program was developed by the guru of keeping track, Daniel Kirschenbaum, Ph.D., a weight expert who's done a number of studies showing that writing down what they eat can help people lose weight. More than two years later, at the age of fourteen and a half, Shanisha weighs between 165 and 170 pounds and is 5'7½" tall.

Shanisha and her mother attended the FitMatters meetings weekly for one year. These meetings included time for the kids and parents to meet in small groups separately with a psychologist. "We talked about what we did that week and what was a struggle," Shanisha's mom explains.

Participants are asked to record everything they eat, along with the fat grams, in a booklet. Shanisha also chose to record the calories in the foods she ate. (Participants are given reference books so they can look up calories and fat grams in various foods.) The goal is to eat a very low-fat diet that's 1,400 calories or less per day under medical supervision.

To get to know how much she was eating, Shanisha and her mother bought measuring cups and spoons. In the beginning, Shanisha says, she measured everything. Now she just measures certain foods, such as rice, beans, and cereal, because it's harder to "eyeball" portions of those foods.

Shanisha also kept track of her physical activity. Participants in the FitMatters program are supposed to get thirty minutes of exercise each day. They're given step counters and a goal of 10,000 steps per day, achieved through walking and just trying to be more active in their daily lives.

Even though her mother wasn't overweight, she kept records, too. The program's philosophy is that kids are more likely to stick with keeping track if they also see their parents doing it. Although the program asked parents to keep records for just the first month, Shanisha's mother did it for the entire year. To help Shanisha get the recommended number of steps each day, her mom walked with her, too. She also tried recipes from low-fat cookbooks (sold to families at a discount through the program), including *Low-Fat Soul* by Jonell Nash.

Now Shanisha and her mother attend the program just twice a month. Her mother continues to encourage Shanisha and the rest of the family to walk everywhere. She says to her kids, "Why get out the car when we can walk?"

More than two years since starting the program, Shanisha still keeps track of what she eats, how many steps she takes, and how much she exercises, but she does so just three days a week. When I asked her why keeping track helps, she explained, "It makes you stop and think. You can look back and say, 'Wow, I ate that much!' Then you can change what you eat the next day." Her mother adds, "Writing everything down is helpful because people don't know what they're doing and what they're eating. It made Shanisha very aware of how much she was eating. It opened her eyes."

Mrs. B. told me that when they started the program, she'd get up in the morning and fix Shanisha breakfast, along with a bag lunch and snacks for the day. She adds, "We got rid of junk food. Dinner would be prepared before I left for work." When I asked her how she pulled this off as a single parent with seven kids (Shanisha's the oldest), she told me, "All eight of us would sit down at the beginning of the week and decide what we'd eat for our dinners. We wrote it down and kept it on our kitchen bulletin board. This let us know what we'd have to take out of the freezer ahead of time and start to prepare each day." All of the kids got involved in planning meals. The older ones would write down the main meals they were going to have for each day of the week, and the little ones would pick out the desserts, usually made from one of their healthy cookbooks.

Shanisha's family still tries to live this way, and everyone pitches in. When I interviewed Shanisha and her mother, for instance, it was the Saturday night before Easter. I could hear all the pleasant commotion in the background as the rest of the kids helped prepare the next day's feast.

I wondered how Mrs. B., with six other children to care for, has time to organize this effort and go to Shanisha's program with her. She told me, "It's something that Shanisha really wants, so I work my schedule around her. Shanisha needs this support because she doesn't have a father in the household. I want her to know she can depend on me."

Even her mom's sisters are involved. Mrs. B. says, "If I can't go to one of Shanisha's classes, my sister will go, or one of them will watch the kids. It's a whole family effort." Mrs. B.'s mother lives nearby and regularly helps out, too. In fact, Shanisha's grandmother and mother split the cost for membership to a gym where Shanisha works out for several hours a couple of times a week — often with her grandmother.

Aside from a small charge for program materials, the FitMatters program hasn't cost Shanisha's family anything. It was developed specifically for people who can't afford expensive weight loss programs and is largely funded through private foundation grants. Medical expenses were paid by insurance, which also covers a small part of the program's costs.

Although Shanisha's mother glances at her daughter's food diary periodically, the tables have turned a bit. Mrs. B. told me, "Now Shanisha says things to me like 'Mom, you know you shouldn't be eating that. Your metabolism is slowing down now that you're in your thirties!'"

Keeping track of what she eats certainly helps Shanisha stay on track with her weight management efforts. She says, "I've stopped eating junk, and I don't eat fast food much at all anymore." She does, however, treat herself about once a month, usually to some ice cream. When she goes to the mall with her friends, she eats at Subway, most often ordering a sub with turkey or ham and mustard instead of mayonnaise. She usually gets the school lunch, finding that there are healthful options if she looks for them.

Although Shanisha said that she'd like to lose another five to ten pounds, she definitely feels that she's accomplished her goals of being able to wear cuter clothes and to "run, walk, and play" without getting tired. When I asked her how her life has changed, she said, "I have more energy, and I feel better." And then she added just these words: "Shorts! And skirts!"

How the Teens Keep Track

Like Shanisha, many of the teens continue to use at least one of the following methods to keep track, even after losing weight: they write down what they eat; they measure or weigh foods; they count calories, fat grams, and/or carbohydrate grams. Many of them use more than one method. It's clear that different strategies work for different teens or work for the same teen at different points in time.

When Jon M. was losing 82 pounds more than five years ago at the age of sixteen, he'd usually write down what he ate right before he went to bed. He says, "Doing it once a day let me think of it more as record keeping for my body—just like I'd make sure my bank account was in order. I allowed myself to eat pretty freely during the day, paying attention to the serving size and trying to eat healthier foods. By writing things down, I could evaluate my day to make sure I was making good choices." Jon also kept track of the minutes of exercise he did each day and how he felt the day went. Once a week, he'd weigh himself and write that down, too.

According to psychologist Nancy Sherwood, Ph.D., a researcher with the HealthPartners Research Foundation in Minneapolis who studies adolescents, self-monitoring strategies are critical for overweight young people who want to arrive and stay at a healthier weight. She notes that there's a wide range of options for exactly what information to record and how often, from keeping a daily record of weight, exercise, and the number of calories and fat grams eaten to recording a general description of foods eaten and exercise each day, with weight recorded weekly or even monthly. The key, she says, is for teens to find some way to track their weight, activity, and eating to help them stay on course without becoming too obsessive.

Why Keeping Track Matters

As Shanisha and her mother pointed out, keeping track helps teens become aware of how much and how often they're eating, as well as how much activity they're getting. Jon M. says, "Keeping a food and exercise diary at first helps you to get an understanding of habits and see what needs to be changed." As pointed out earlier, Jon's record keeping also helped him track his progress and stay "honest" with himself. Xavier L. religiously wrote down everything he ate in a food diary, measured foods, and kept track of the "points" he ate on his Weight Watchers plan while he was losing weight. He says, "This gave me an element of control over my life."

Ally S., who lost 56 pounds five years ago, found that keeping a food and exercise diary helped her identify patterns that were tripping her up. She explains, "If I didn't lose any weight, I might look back on the week and see that I'd eaten out a lot. Or if I saw that I didn't work out much, it explained why my clothes were fitting differently. Writing things down helped me with self-assessment."

Although only a handful of studies have been conducted on self-monitoring in teens, virtually every expert I consulted feels that keeping track is an important tool for overweight teens who want to get to a healthier weight. (And a growing body of research indicates that it helps adults lose weight, too.) Brian Saelens, Ph.D., of Cincinnati Children's Hospital Medical Center headed one study on self-monitoring in a small group of overweight twelve- to sixteen-year-olds. The kids were encouraged to write down all the foods and beverages they consumed daily, noting the amount and calorie value of each food. The results showed that the kids who recorded something in their food diaries at least five times per day lost more weight than did those who recorded less diligently.

A more recent study on self-monitoring, by Daniel Kirschenbaum, Ph.D., Julie Germann, Ph.D., and Barry Rich, M.D., published in the journal *Obesity Research*, involved eighty-three obese teens in the Fit-Matters program. The teens who wrote down what they ate on most days lost significantly more weight in the first month of the program than did those who didn't keep track at all. During the third month of the program, only the kids who kept track most of the time lost weight. This study also found that when the teens' parents wrote down what they ate, too, the teens were more likely to do it—and they lost more weight than did the teens whose parents didn't keep track.

Keeping Track of Specifics: Calories, Fat Grams, and Carbs

One out of 4 teens said that they counted calories while they were losing weight. Interestingly, even more of them (36) said that they count calories now, after slimming down. And 23 teens said that they count fat grams. Molly S. says, "When I was losing weight, I wrote down everything, all the time—even a bite of chicken. I counted every calorie in every piece of food I ate—always." Although she's eased up on calorie counting, she says, "still, I usually keep a pretty good count in my head." Given how few teens said that they lost weight by following a low-carb diet, I was surprised to find that almost 1 out of 4 of them said that they count carbs, after having lost weight.

Further questioning revealed that some of the teens who said they *counted* calories, fat grams, or carbs don't actually count them, but are simply aware of the amount of each in various foods. For instance, Xavier L. said that he counts carbohydrate grams. But when I asked him to tell me more about this, he said that he tries to limit his intake of simple carbohydrates from foods such as sweets. He explains, "I do eat carbs and do not rigorously count grams, but I'm conscious of the proportion of carbs to what else I'm eating." Similarly, Jorgey W., who indicated on

Making Tracks

Keeping a simple food diary, noting the types and amounts of foods and beverages consumed, is the tracking activity that probably helps most with weight management. Options for keeping track run the gamut from blank notebooks and checkbook registers to special journals designed for weight management to computer programs and special Web sites.

A daily record might look something like the following list. Additional columns could be added to record calories and fat grams. Other categories might include mood, weight, degree of hunger, and/or physical activity.

Morning:
- 1 banana
- 1 cup skim milk
- 1 cup Cheerios

Lunchtime:
- Turkey sandwich: 2 slices rye bread, 3 slices turkey breast, 1 slice provolone cheese, 1 tablespoon low-fat mayo
- 1 medium apple
- 1-ounce bag of baked chips
- 8-ounce carton of low-fat chocolate milk

After school:
- 2 long pretzel sticks
- 2 pieces of string cheese
- 1 handful of popcorn
- 1 plum

Suppertime:
- 4 ounces meat loaf
- 1 medium baked potato with 2 tablespoons low-fat sour cream
- 1 cup green beans
- 2 cups tossed salad
- 3 tablespoons low-fat Italian dressing
- 1 cup skim milk

After supper:
- 1 cup vanilla frozen yogurt
- 3 tablespoons fat-free chocolate sauce

Physical activity:
- Rollerbladed for 30 minutes.
- Took stairs instead of elevator twice.
- Walked home from school instead of getting a ride.

her questionnaire that she counts fat grams and calories, told me that she just "looks at them" on food labels.

Some experts who run weight programs told me that they recommend counting for selected teens only. Kerri Boutelle, Ph.D., an expert in adolescent weight and eating disorders at the University of Minnesota, says, "We tend not to have kids count calories because it's usually not very accurate. If we have a teen who likes math, however, we might have him or her count them." She has also conducted some studies on self-monitoring with Dr. Daniel Kirschenbaum and concludes, "Detailed recording of calories, fat grams, or carbs is not necessary for most teens. What's important is trying to write down what you eat most of the time."

Weighing and Measuring Foods

When I asked Nicole S., who's lost almost 150 pounds and kept it off for about two years, to list the three most important things she does to maintain her weight loss, number one on the list was "I make sure that I weigh and measure my foods." She also keeps a food diary every day. Similarly, when Xavier L. was losing weight, he measured everything "except nonstarchy vegetables."

There's no question that the best way to determine portion size is to do what these teens did. How else does someone know exactly what half a cup of pasta or four ounces of meat looks like on a dinner plate, or how much one-half cup of ice cream really is?

As portion sizes became familiar, the teens often eased up. Shanisha B., Ally S., and Xavier L. told me that now they weigh only certain foods — such as pasta, rice, and cold cereal — if it's hard to judge the portion size by eye.

Keeping Track — but Not Going Crazy

Keeping track doesn't have to involve anything fancy (see page 163). What's most important is for each teen to find a method of recording that's convenient for him or her. Wes G. and Jon M. both used a daily planner — a small, booklet-type calendar with blank spaces for the days of the week.

The best plan is to keep track throughout the day, as Shanisha B. does. She says, "My friends know, and no one gives me a hard time about it. If someone asks me what I'm doing, I just tell them." Some teens don't feel comfortable keeping track so visibly. Writing things down at the end of the day is okay, too.

Wilson S. advises, "Keep track at times when you're bored. I did it on the computer during my computer classes or my free classes." Ally S. keeps a little notepad beside her computer so she can keep rough track of how many calories she's eaten each day.

Record keeping can become obsessive for some teens. Paula D. says, "Obsessing by counting calories and weighing food is the worst for me." Ally S. says, "Keeping track of your food and your exercise could just mean writing a few notes on a piece of paper. It's important to give yourself 'free days' where you don't write anything down." She told me that she has eased up on all the tracking she did while losing weight.

Although some experts think it's too hard for teens to record everything they eat, day in and day out, Dr. Daniel Kirschenbaum believes that a "healthy obsession" is in order for overweight teens and adults alike who want to lose weight and keep it off. Record keeper Nicole S. makes no bones about the difficulty: "You have to be strong, because it takes a lot of work, and sometimes it's hard."

Dr. Kerri Boutelle says that many overweight people are not attentive enough and that "the idea is to get them to focus more on what they're eating." She notes, however, that her program determines who should keep records on an individual basis. "If we have a teen who's very anxious, obsessive, and critical of herself, we would probably not have her write down what she eats."

KEEPING TRACK THEN AND NOW

Some of the teens said that they don't find it necessary to keep track as rigorously now as in the beginning. Jon M., who wrote down everything when he was losing, says, "I have graduated to keeping just a mental checklist as I go through the day — paying attention to what I'm eating, along with the amount of exercise I'm getting."

Jorgey W., who lost more than 100 pounds, wrote down everything she ate and drank every day and counted "every calorie and fat gram" while she was losing weight. Now, she says, "I just watch what I eat, and I look things up only occasionally." Other teens echoed this sentiment, saying that they do these things now only under certain circumstances. For instance, Xavier L. usually just keeps a mental note of what he eats but "rigorously journals when things get out of control." Molly S. says, "Now I only count calories and record everything when I'm trying to get ready for a big event such as the prom."

Weighing In

Many of the teens have discovered that weighing themselves on a regular basis is another important way to keep track. Shanisha B. weighs herself whenever she attends the FitMatters program—twice a month now, but weekly in the beginning. She told me that she doesn't get anxious about stepping on the scale. In fact, she says, "I want to weigh in. If my weight is up, I don't get upset; I just try to figure out why."

When I asked the teens, "How do you know how much you weigh?" more than 8 out of 10 said that they weigh themselves on a scale. A small number said that they go just by the fit of their clothing. A little more than a quarter of the teens (28) weigh themselves once a week, 22 do so more than once a week, 19 weigh themselves once or twice a month, and just 5 weigh themselves only when they go to the doctor's office or every couple of months. (Only some of the teens answered this question.) Similarly, the National Weight Control Registry has found that most formerly overweight adults weigh themselves regularly.

Adolescent weight experts disagree about how often teens should weigh themselves when trying to lose weight. Shelley Kirk, Ph.D., R.D., director of the HealthWorks! program for kids at Cincinnati Children's Hospital Medical Center, says that the program checks participants' weight only every two or three weeks. She doesn't recommend that kids weigh themselves between visits because the program focuses on behavioral changes to improve eating habits and physical activity rather than on a specific weight goal. However, there's some limited evidence that more frequent weighing results in greater weight losses, at least over the short term.

Most of the experts I interviewed said that the teens in their programs weigh in once a week. Adolescent weight expert Thomas Robinson, M.D., of Stanford University says, "Some kids can get obsessed with the daily ups and/or downs of the numbers on the scale and miss the greater importance of following longer-term trends over time." Also, because most scales are not sensitive enough to detect day-to-day changes in weight, daily weighing can be discouraging or even misleading.

Dr. Nancy Sherwood concludes, "There's not a one-size-fits-all answer to the question about how often teens should weigh themselves. Daily, weekly, or even monthly self-monitoring of weight may work for different teens at different times. Ideally, teens can get to a place where the weight on the scale is not an indicator of their self-worth and does not determine their mood for the day but rather can be used as feedback about their weight management program."

Nipping Small Weight Gains in the Bud

The teens have found it easier to lose a small amount of weight than to gain back 20 or 30 pounds and have to start all over again. Zach G. says that one of the most important things he does to keep the weight off is "if I gain five pounds, I immediately lose it. I do something right away." Likewise, McKenzie K. says, "I can always tell if my pants have gotten tighter or if I weigh more. Then I know it's time to watch what I eat or work out more."

Some teens mentioned that if they gain a little weight, the first thing they do is try to determine why this happened. Katie S. says, "I try to figure out what changed in my life." Taylor S. says, "I identify my dietary weakness and address it." If Shanisha B. gains, she exercises more, counts calories and fat grams, keeps a food diary, and cuts back on snacks and sweets. College track team member Tyler D., who keeps his weight within a ten-pound range, says, "I have to eat a lot during track season, but then I have to readjust when it's over. When I went home last summer, I noticed I was gaining weight, so I started running again. If my weight's up, I also cut back on snacking and drink more water."

Here are the teens' most common responses to my question "What do you do if you start to gain back some weight?" The top four responses were mentioned by more than half of the teens, way ahead of all the others. Most of the teens gave multiple responses. (An equal number of teens gave the last two responses.)

1. Exercise more.
2. Give up or cut back on snacks.
3. Give up or cut back on sweets.
4. Decrease portions.
5. Count calories.
6. Go on a diet.
7. Keep a food diary.
8. Count fat grams.
9. Go back to person or group that helped me lose.
10. Count carbs.

Setting Realistic Goals

The teens' stories illustrate over and over that one of the ways to shift the focus away from the scale and toward habits that can more directly be controlled is to set small, easily achievable goals. "I often got discouraged when I failed to meet my lofty goals, like 'I'm giving up ice cream,'" my son Wes says. "I succeeded when I used landmarks like 'I'll only have ice cream once a week.'"

Paula D. says, "I decided to break down the scary lifestyle change I knew I needed to make into smaller, more manageable changes." Margaret G. lost about 25 pounds between the ages of sixteen and twenty-one by making small changes. She stopped adding gravy to foods, ate fewer sweets, took smaller portions, and continued to be active in sports, bike riding, and a dance group.

Parents can help teens set goals that are achievable in reasonable amounts of time; are measurable, not vague; and are reasonable, not perfectionistic. Examples might include having breakfast five mornings a week, spending no more than two hours a day in front of the TV or

What's a Parent's Role in Keeping Track?

As with every other strategy in this book, the initiative for keeping track has to come from the teen. Dr. Nancy Sherwood says, "Parents can explain the rationale for self-monitoring—that it's just a tool to help them stay on track. Parents can also help teens figure out what monitoring strategies are right for them." But it's up to the teen to follow through. Parents can ask whether they'd like to have gentle reminders to do so.

Parents who are keeping track along with their teen might compare notes and discuss how they're doing, but in a noncompetitive way. Certainly, parents should never use teens' records in a judgmental or critical way. Kids need to be praised for the very fact that they're keeping track.

Dr. Sherwood emphasizes that parents can also help teens look at their records matter-of-factly, as data that will help them be more aware of what they're eating and how they might change. Teens who want input might find it helpful for parents to go over their food and exercise diaries with them to help them identify what might be getting in the way of their efforts and come up with solutions to problems. Perhaps the family has too many sweets around or gets take-out food too often. Maybe the family eats too much in the evening and could go for a walk or play games together instead. Of course, the best way to identify problems and come up with solutions when keeping track is to work with a health care professional, such as a registered dietitian, who's skilled in this area.

As for weighing in, what the scale says is a private matter, to be shared only if the teen wants to. Again, the information should never be used in a critical way. Rather, it should be used simply to determine how well a plan is working and whether to make changes when the teen gets stuck.

playing video games, or having fast food no more than once a week. The teens can then keep track of their progress. If a goal doesn't seem achievable, it should be adjusted.

How the Teens Reward Themselves

Some teens told me that they give themselves rewards for their accomplishments. Parents can help, but only if the teen wants it that way and the reward system is set up together. Molly S.'s mother told me that some of the rewards they came up with as Molly was losing weight were allowing her to have a sleepover, to go on a shopping trip, or to get her hair colored.

Ally S. says that for each five or ten pounds she lost, she'd treat herself to something like a new outfit, some new accessories, or a new pair of shoes. "They can be small rewards," she explains, "but just acknowledging success in some way really helps to keep you motivated."

It's normal for teens to reward themselves for pounds lost, but it's also important to reward themselves for meeting other goals—ones they can directly control and achieve. For example, if a teen keeps a food journal for ten days out of a two-week stretch, he could reward himself with a new CD or by going to a movie. Or if a teen meets her exercise goals for a week, she could reward herself with some new jewelry or a magazine. Obviously, using food as a reward for weight loss defeats the purpose.

Simply reminding themselves of the benefits of arriving at a healthier weight is itself rewarding. Aaron T. says, "There are the compliments from everyone, being able to fit into a medium shirt and looking skinny as can be. And girls—I didn't have the guts to ask a girl out before, but losing weight helped me get the confidence to get a girlfriend. This, if nothing else, should motivate teens."

8

Tuning In
Putting Mind and Body Together

> I used to eat anything and everything I could get my
> hands on, regardless of my hunger level. Now I focus
> on healthy foods and listen to my hunger. — **Marie P.**

The teens reported that they have figured out how to tune in to their
hunger signals and their emotions, so their eating is more in line with
their bodies' needs. And when they "slip" from the course they've charted,
they talk to themselves in positive terms that get them back on track.

JEANA S.'S STORY

"My weight loss journey began when I was in the eighth grade," Jeana S.
told me the first time we spoke. "I lost 12 pounds between eighth and
tenth grades. By exercising and eating mindfully, I kept my weight at
around 140 for the rest of my high school years. Then, when I was a
sophomore in college, I lost another 10 pounds. It's made a huge difference in my life." Jeana started out weighing 152 pounds, and she's held
her weight steady at 130 for about two years. (Throughout all this time,
her height has remained 5'3".)

When I asked Jeana the most important thing she did to lose
weight, she said, "I started paying attention to what I put in my mouth."
She also learned to deal with her emotions without turning to food for
comfort. In short, she used her head to get a handle on her weight —
and she still does.

Jeana says that her weight gain was the result of "a lot of little things that added up" as she went from thirteen to fifteen. She was always active in sports—volleyball, cheerleading, and cross-country—but during middle school, she started spending more of her at-home time doing schoolwork than helping out on the dairy farm her parents owned. She says, "I put pressure on myself to do well in school. So I'd stay up until 1:00 or 2:00 A.M. doing homework. And when you stay up late, you get hungry. So I'd eat huge bowlfuls of cereal at midnight. I also ate a lot socially with friends. I'd get a soda pop or juice drink along with a snack because that's what my friends were doing, not because I was hungry." Jeana feels that school lunches were part of the problem. "The portions were just too big, and many of the foods weren't the best for your weight." She also recalls having a crush on a guy who had a daily habit of getting candy and a Mountain Dew from the school's vending machines. She started doing that, too, to get his attention.

When she reached puberty, Jeana figured "some weight gain was inevitable," but she vowed that she'd "never top 150 pounds." When she hit 152, she says, "I knew it was time to do something." After a few "crazy" diets left her feeling disgusted, Jeana tried the "exercise only" approach. That didn't help her lose weight either, because, she says, "I continued to pretty much eat whatever I wanted."

The turning point came at the end of eighth grade, when Jeana spent a week visiting an older cousin who got her hooked on walking. Jeana says, "My cousin and her family also ate very well—lots of fresh veggies, served wonderfully, and a lot of low-fat foods. It was then that I made the connection that eating and exercising have to go hand in hand." This discovery was bolstered by things she read in *Prevention* and *Vitality*, two magazines lying around her house. She says, "They both offered great advice and information to support my new approach to weight loss, which was basically eating unprocessed foods, having six mini-meals a day, packing my own lunch, and following the food guide pyramid." When I pointed out that this was rather a heady way for a fifteen-year-old to go about things, Jeana said, "I was very mature at a young age. I had an unquenchable thirst for knowledge, and I read all I could about weight loss."

Jeana also took a great deal of initiative in ensuring that she got the foods she needed and wanted. She explains, "We rarely ate together as a family; we just fed ourselves. If I wanted healthy foods in the house, it was up to me." Before she learned to drive, she'd give her mom a list of food requests when her mom went shopping. In the morning, she'd typically have oatmeal, a glass of skim milk, and a little beef jerky or lean sausage made from their own farm animals. The night before, she'd pack a mid-morning snack and lunch for the next day: carrots, skim milk, and dry cereal. At lunchtime, her home economics teachers allowed Jeana to use the microwave oven to zap her favorite combination—RyKrisp crackers topped with tuna and melted cheese. Along with the cracker combination, she might have vegetable soup and a container of skim milk, which she bought in the cafeteria. After school—before or after sports practices—a typical snack would be a piece of fruit and some frozen peas that she kept in the home ec freezer. For dinner, she might fix herself baked fish, a vegetable, a microwaved potato, and a glass of skim milk. "Slowly," she says, "the pounds came off, and I felt great."

For the next six months or so, Jeana would eat whatever she brought to school, whether she was hungry for it or not. But the next fall, when she was in ninth grade, the "mindfulness" part of her weight journey came into play at the suggestion of her school nurse, who noticed Jeana's weight loss efforts when she went into the nurse's office to weigh in on the scale. Jeana says, "The nurse gave me some food journal sheets that had spaces for recording what, how much, and why I ate. She said it wasn't the detailed record keeping that mattered so much as starting to pay attention to what and why I was eating. It helped me become more thoughtful about what I was doing. I started really tuning in to what I was eating—feeling the shredded wheat or smelling the apple. I also paid more attention to hunger, being full, and why I was eating. If I started to get full when eating a meal, I'd leave a piece of food behind."

Playing at Being Full

A fascinating study on teaching children to tune in to their hunger signals, published in *Pediatrics,* involved a small group of preschoolers who ranged from being underweight to being overweight. Some were overeaters, some didn't eat enough, and others ate appropriate amounts of food for their weight. At the outset, the researchers found that the heavier kids and the kids whose mothers were dieters and impulsive eaters were less likely to eat according to their bodies' needs than were the children of mothers without these tendencies.

For the study, the children attended a six-week program in which the researchers performed skits with themes centering on rumbling in the stomach (to represent hunger), eating until full, and signals associated with overeating, such as stomach discomfort. The kids also watched and discussed the videotape *Winnie the Pooh and the Honey Tree* and played with specially made dolls with tummies of varying degrees of fullness to help them identify cues of hunger and fullness.

After the program, both undereaters and overeaters had improved their ability to focus on internal cues of hunger and satisfaction, and they ate accordingly. Furthermore, their eating was no longer related to their mothers' eating habits. After several weeks, when the researchers would prompt the kids during snack time to tune in and see how hungry or full they were, they began saying things such as "I'm not hungry anymore, so I'm going to stop eating" or "My stomach's getting full." The researchers concluded that the program helped both finicky eaters, who previously didn't eat enough in response to hunger cues, and heavier children, who tended to eat more than their bodies needed, to learn how to eat more appropriate amounts of food for their weight.

The author of the study, Susan Johnson, Ph.D., of the University of Colorado Health Sciences Center, says, "Having conversations with children of all ages about what hunger and fullness feel like should help them maintain healthy body weights and a healthy relationship with food and eating."

Jeana also tuned in to her pace of eating. She noticed that at the beginning of a meal, when she was really hungry, she would eat faster than toward the end of the meal. So when she saw herself slowing down, she started asking herself, "Am I just continuing [to eat] out of habit? Have I met my body's needs?" She still does this.

The final part of putting her head and her body together was tackling her tendency to eat when she was emotionally upset. In fact, Jeana's decision to do something about her weight was partly spurred by the ridicule she suffered from her peers, even though she was not as overweight as many of the other teens I spoke with. She says, "Before I lost weight, I had very large breasts for my age, and kids used to tease me about them endlessly. It hurt a lot, and I used food to calm the feelings. And I often ate when I was lonely or stressed."

She learned how to handle her emotions without turning to food while attending a camp to learn how to be a peer helper. There teens were taught how to get in touch with their emotions by keeping a journal. Today, when Jeana feels like eating for an emotional reason, she still writes about her feelings in a journal. Or she might talk to a friend or to her dad, with whom she's always had a close relationship. If she feels lonely, she calls a friend or grabs a book. Finally, she says, "I might exercise. It clears the slate, clears my brain, and gives me the physical boost to ride through the rocky times and celebrate the good times."

After Jeana went off to college, she lost 10 more pounds by stepping up the intensity of her exercise and doing it more regularly. She also stopped eating after eight o'clock in the evening and avoided alcohol. She says, "There's definitely a family tendency to be heavy, and I think that by losing weight when I did, I headed off a problem that could have become much bigger." She's twenty-two now and admits that maintaining her weight takes effort. She says, "It would be much easier to eat without thinking and just sit around. But I'd feel like crap." Managing her weight has gotten easier with time, she says, and the effort is worth the payback: "I like the way I feel and look right now, and that helps me stay motivated."

TUNING IN TO THE BODY'S HUNGER SIGNALS

Like Jeana S., many of the teens said that they used to eat without thinking and to continue to eat after they were full. My son was like that. At a Fourth of July celebration when Wes was about nine, he devoured eleven cupcakes "to be funny." Another time, he won a pizza-eating contest by downing a large deep-dish pepperoni pizza in eight minutes. He once told me that he had no mechanism to tell him when to stop eating. Now, however, he can leave food on his plate, even if it's one of his favorites. When I asked how he found the "mechanism" that tells him when to stop eating, he replied, "I listened for it and looked for it and eventually taught myself to recognize it. I learned to recognize that maybe I could still eat more but that I didn't need it." He also said that he sometimes asks himself if he'd rather have the extra food as fat on his body or in the trash can.

Many of the other teens, like Ethan A. and Felicia S., learned to tune in to their body's hunger signals, too.

Ethan Q.

Then: "I used to be so hungry in my mind that I'd keep eating and eating. But there was never time for my body to get the message that I was full, so I'd eat some more. I'd sit around my house and try to amuse myself, but I always found myself in front of the pantry. It was like a constant hunger whenever I was bored, even though I knew that I wasn't really hungry."

Now: "I know I'm hungry when my stomach feels kind of empty and I feel hunger pangs. I eat until I satisfy the empty feeling, not until I'm uncomfortable and can't eat anymore."

Felicia S.

Then: "I didn't eat regular meals. I just ate when I felt like eating. And when I was full, I'd still keep eating."

Now: "I know I'm hungry when my stomach is growling. But I don't just go by my stomach growling, because sometimes it growls *after* I eat. Another thing that helps me is to be on a routine—eating breakfast, lunch, and dinner. I put only normal-size portions on my plate so I'm not tempted to keep eating when I'm satisfied. I also ask myself why I feel like eating—is it because I'm bored or truly hungry?"

When Mindful Eating Needs a Little Help

Sometimes it's just plain hard to eat only when hungry and stop when full. The teens use some tricks that help them eat more mindfully.

They slow down. Ethan Q. says, "Slowing down when I eat gives my stomach time to catch up to what I'm eating." Sometimes waiting twenty minutes or so helps a person decide whether he or she is truly hungry.

They brush their teeth. McKenzie K. says, "Brush your teeth after you eat or when you feel you've eaten enough. This keeps me from eating more, because I don't want to brush again."

They chew gum. Aaron T. says, "The best way for me to stop the munchies is to chew gum—the sugar-free kind, of course. I always used to want something in my mouth, so I used gum as a way to stop my cravings."

They do something else. Marie P. learned new habits in place of going to the cookie jar when she got home from school: "I started having a piece of fruit and going for a run instead." Now if she feels the temptation to keep eating after a meal, she says, "I usually find something to occupy myself—like painting my nails, going for a walk, or calling a friend to talk. Usually, by the time I've finished, I'm no longer hungry or thinking about going back to the kitchen."

They get enough sleep. Aaron T. says, "Having the discipline to get enough sleep is critical for losing weight." Recent research indicates that he's onto something. A growing number of studies suggest that sleep deprivation may play a role in overeating and becoming overweight. Part of the reason for this appears to be that lack of sleep causes shifts in hormones that influence hunger and appetite. People who are awake for more hours also have more time to think about food and to eat than do people who sleep more. According to MayoClinic.com, nine hours of sleep a night is optimal for teens.

They avoid things that trigger eating. Ben G. tries not to open the cupboards and refrigerator. Aaron T. stays out of the kitchen as much as possible.

GETTING A HANDLE ON EMOTIONAL OVEREATING

Like Jeana S., other teens have learned to get a handle on emotional eating.

My son Wes says, "Emotional overeating was definitely one of the initial causes of my weight gain. Eating felt good, so I ate in response to any emotion — boredom, anger, loneliness. But I made a conscious decision to stop doing this. When I had an urge to eat, I'd ask myself why that was. Then I found other outlets for my emotions — shooting hoops was a good way to get out anger or aggression. When I was lonely, I'd call a friend. Now rather than eat when I'm bored, I might do origami or throw a Frisbee to my dog." When Ally S. wants to eat for emotional reasons, she might run on her treadmill or use a boxing bag.

Eating for emotional reasons was partly responsible for Felicia S.'s weight gain, which started at age seven or eight, when her parents were going through a divorce. Shortly thereafter, her mother died. She says, "Now when I look back, food was one of the few things I enjoyed at the time, and I'm sure I ate to push my thoughts away." She discovered that "eating for emotional reasons doesn't work because it only makes you feel better for a short time."

Just recently, Felicia had to remind herself of this when she found herself turning to food because of schoolwork. "I had to reteach myself not to eat when stressed-out at school. I remembered how people say that when you exercise, your body makes endorphins, the chemicals that help you feel better. I didn't believe it, but I found out it was true when I started exercising again. Exercise helps me more than eating does."

Several teens said that keeping a journal is a good way to channel emotions, and a number of them find that it helps to talk with a friend or other supportive person. Jeana S. says, "I turned to my diary and my dad."

Katie S. admits that she used to overeat to get back at her mother. She explains, "My mom was always trying to control me, and I wanted to show her that I was in control of my own life. The one thing I could use to get under her skin was to eat, because she didn't want me to be overweight." Katie recalls going with her family to a local deli one Friday night. She intended to eat just half of an overstuffed sandwich and save the rest for another time. But after her mother said, "Why do you need to eat that?" she ate the whole thing just to make her mom mad. She says, "I now see that eating to get back at someone is actually taking my power away from me. I never got anything from it, and I kept gaining more weight."

Some teens still struggle with eating for emotional reasons or eating out of boredom. Christine F. says, "Sometimes I give in to it. It's okay to eat ice cream over the kitchen sink when feeling horrible—just so it's a monthly situation or less frequent." Katie S. adds, "There are times when I want to eat because I'm bored. But since I know I'm doing that, I'll try to find things that don't have a lot of consequences, like carrots, popcorn, or oatmeal."

MOVING ON FROM SLIPS

The teens do slip, of course, but they've learned how to prevent lapses from becoming full-blown relapses. Only two of the teens made comments about giving up and continuing to eat when they slip.

Jeana S. says that when she overate, "I'd tell myself that I was going to be okay, even though I'd lost control momentarily. I'd write this in my journal and add self-praise, like 'Jeana, you're doing really good overall. This isn't the end of the world.' Then I'd stay out of the kitchen for a little while and get back on track."

When I looked at Jeana's and other teens' responses to my question about slipping, I realized that many of them use what's called "positive self-talk." Katie S. says that when she eats too many of her favorite honey-mustard pretzels, instead of telling herself "I'm a failure" and going overboard the rest of the day, she asks herself, "Am I going to gain

How the Teens
Recover After a Slip

They write it off and start over. Sid J. thinks, "Tomorrow is a new day, with a chance of a new beginning."

They make an adjustment later on. Mike D. says, "I let it go and just ease up at the next meal."

They put it in perspective. Paula D. says, "Sometimes I eat fattening foods like cookie batter and feel guilty. When that happens, I decide to look at the situation rationally. It's one slip-up, and it's not really that big of a deal. It's not like I'm going to gain five pounds just because I ate a lot of cookie batter. Plus, I figure that everyone needs a cookie batter day once in a while."

They exercise to offset it. If Paula D. has a "cookie batter day," she might add a day of exercise so that she works out four days that week instead of three. She adds, "But I *do not* over–work out. In other words, I make sure that I do not try to overcompensate for a momentary lapse in judgment."

They figure out why it happened. Taylor S. says, "If I slip, I can't hold it over my head. Once it's done, it's done. Instead of hounding myself, I try to find out why it happened. Then I try to figure out what I need to do to avoid it in the future."

weight from that one incident? That can be my one treat for the day." She applies the same strategy when she slacks off on exercise. "When I missed two weeks of doing sit-ups, I felt the loss of muscle tone in my stomach. I could have said, 'I may as well not bother doing them anymore.' Instead, I said to myself, 'Missing sit-ups for two weeks doesn't mean my whole body contour is going to change. It's not the end of my success.'"

Even if some slipping here and there leads to a bit of weight gain, the teens don't turn it into a catastrophe. When Richie C. gained back a little weight, he at first felt like a failure, then he rallied. "I realized that it was only a few pounds, not a major setback. I just needed to buckle down and focus on a healthy lifestyle." Katie S. says, "There will always be little blips in time. A lapse does not mean the end of my success."

9
Staying Pumped
Remaining Motivated to Keep the Weight Off

> Every time I start leaning back toward the overweight side, I simply change my lifestyle to make sure I don't return to the person I once was. **— Tyler D.**

It's one thing to arrive at a just-right weight; it's another to stay there. How do the teens get themselves to keep doing the things that work? How do they stay pumped to keep the weight off?

DAVID G.'S STORY

David G. responded to an ad I placed in his college newspaper. He told me that from tenth through twelfth grades, he lost 65 pounds by "overall healthy eating—with moderation of 'bad' foods—along with exercise and avoiding eating at night." I was particularly intrigued when he said, "Although it all seemed incredibly difficult, I'd have to say that the physical aspect of losing weight was only about half the battle. Not getting discouraged and keeping myself motivated was just as hard."

The most important thing he did to maintain his momentum for three years, as well as to keep the weight off, was to change his lifestyle. "Instead of going on diets and failing, I started making changes I could live with for the rest of my life. It was a change in my mindset." Today, as a college sophomore, David weighs 195 pounds—down from his all-time high of 260—and is a muscular 5'11", two inches taller than he was at his heaviest.

David started gaining excess weight when he was about eight, mainly because of lack of exercise, too much TV watching, and excessive snacking. He decided to slim down because he was tired of being ostracized and wanted his clothes to fit right. The real clincher was that he wanted to have a girlfriend. "I decided to do whatever it takes," he says. "I'd look at food and ask myself, 'What's more important—having this extra serving of something or getting in shape?'"

David learned the hard way that going to extremes didn't work. "I looked at my failures from the past, like the Atkins diet, and realized that as soon as I went off the diet, the weight came back on. The same thing happened when I'd try to lose weight by eating one meal a day or cutting back too far on calories, as I did one year when I was on the wrestling team. I saw that I couldn't just go on a diet."

When David finally succeeded, he started out on his own by "taking little steps," such as giving up regular soda and unhealthful snacks. For instance, he'd try some vegetables he hadn't had in a while or eat carrots with fat-free ranch dressing instead of chips. He says, "I was doing things I liked, just different things." David also did some experimenting. For instance, in the beginning, he ate only vegetables and lean meats for a week or two. He soon discovered that "it was too much at once. I realized that if I cut out things that I really enjoyed, I'd crave them. So it became important to have these things, but in moderation." Take peanut butter, which he loves. He allowed himself to have a peanut butter sandwich one or two days a week. "Finding that balance was important," he says.

David is one of the few teens who said he followed a low-carbohydrate diet. When I asked him for the details, however, it turned out that although he cut back on the amount of pasta, bread, and sweets he'd been eating previously, he didn't really follow a strict low-carb diet. He told me, "I'd eat carbs throughout the day—fruits, veggies, and bread —especially if I was going to be doing a lot of cardio exercise that day." David also ate fewer high-fat foods and switched to low-fat and fat-free versions of many products, such as milk and ice cream. And he found it helpful to eat five or six small meals a day rather than a few larger ones.

During high school, David lived with his aunt and uncle, who were not overweight but tended to serve fattening foods and have snacks such as cookies and fudge around the house. Nevertheless, they praised David's efforts and were willing to buy and make him foods that helped with his quest to achieve a healthier weight. Slowly, he noticed that their eating habits started changing for the better, too.

At the same time that he was making all these dietary changes, David says, he realized that "watching TV didn't do it for me anymore." He slowly began to jog, one-half mile at a time, and lift weights several times a week at a local gym. Eventually, his runs became longer, and he added workouts on a stair-climber, stationary bicycle, or elliptical machine.

In addition to changing his eating habits and activities, David came up with a number of motivational strategies. He found it helpful to tell people around him what he wanted to accomplish in his weight loss efforts. He says, "The more people you tell, the more likely you are to succeed." He also made a list of things he looked forward to doing when he was in shape, such as looking good without a shirt on. For incentive, he'd sometimes buy a shirt that was a bit too small and hang it in his room.

"Taking things day by day," he gave himself a daily score from 1 to 10 on a calendar, based on how he felt he'd done for the day when it came to eating and exercise. "If I didn't eat any fried foods or too many sweets and I got a good run in, I'd get a higher score." Then, at the end of the week, he looked for patterns. "At one point, I noticed I was getting 8s and 9s on weekdays but 3s and 4s on the weekends. This showed me where I needed to improve. It also gave me perspective. I saw that a not-so-great weekend wasn't going to hurt me, because I was still making progress."

David attributes much of his success to getting into a routine. "A lot of it was getting used to what I was doing and accepting that things weren't going to happen overnight. I really started seeing it as a process —not just reaching a number on the scale." Although the eating and activity changes were critical to his success, David says that a shift in his mindset needed to occur to make the change happen and to make it last.

Now that he's down to a comfortable weight, David's eating habits haven't changed too much from the time when he was losing. He still does best when he tries not to go overboard with carbs, includes plenty of lean protein (such as skinless chicken), watches his fat intake, and mentally keeps track of what he eats each day. About once a week, he feeds his sweet tooth, "usually by having a little ice cream and not worrying about it."

David is quite the athlete now and plays on his college racquetball team. He also does some toning exercises and sometimes runs or goes for hikes.

He acknowledges that he's "slipped back a few times," including when he first went to college and started eating at the school cafeteria. "I gained the 'freshman fifteen' and thought to myself, 'Am I going to lose this weight or stay the same?' I knew I couldn't just 'go on a diet,' so I took steps that would help me lose the extra weight. I allowed myself to go through the cafeteria line only once, ate slower, and had a glass of water before my meal, plus a glass of milk with my meal."

David stays motivated by keeping a picture of himself at his highest weight on his refrigerator and thinking of how he felt then. But he doesn't use it in a punishing way. "Once I developed a healthy lifestyle, I saw it as a challenge, and now I enjoy it. I don't have to do this; I do this because it's who I am." (And, yes, he got a girlfriend.)

THE TEENS REMEMBER THE PAST

The main way the teens stay motivated is the way David G. does: they keep a vivid picture — figurative, literal, or both — of themselves when they were heavier, and they think about how they don't want to go back to that life. Zach G. says, "I look at old photos and say, 'I can't go back to that.' I was known as 'Big Zach,' but now people say I'm skinny. When I lost weight, I felt like a new person. That keeps me motivated. Also, I'm afraid of being treated the old way again." Jorgey W. has a photo on her fridge, along with a sign that says NOTHING TASTES AS GOOD AS BEING THIN FEELS. Missy S. went so far as to make a quilt from her old jeans and says, "It reminds me of all my hard work."

Other teens never forget their pasts either. Taylor S. says, "The thought of being overweight again is enough to keep me in check. I stay at it by simply remembering how far I've come." Mary N. adds, "I keep doing the things I did to lose weight because I know that if I don't, I'll feel the way I did before I lost the weight. I just think of where I was and how far I've come. It was too much work to turn back." Tyler D. agrees, saying, "My body was fat, and it wants to be fat again. So I get pissed off at it and don't allow it to happen."

They Focus on the Payback

The teens don't just focus on the past to stay motivated — they recognize the payback of being at a healthier weight. What keeps Nicole K. motivated is the confidence she's gained since losing more than 65 pounds. She says, "I'm just a happier person." Eleck F.'s method of staying psyched is to "look in the mirror — that's all the motivation I need." After a trip to Mexico, Amber M., who has kept off about 150 pounds for more than a decade, told me, "It felt really wonderful to be the most beautiful blonde on the beach. I never thought I would have said that twelve years ago!" Vincent J. says, "I love the attention from all the girls I know. When I was fat, no girl would look at me." Paula D. stays psyched by the tank tops she can wear now — ones that show her arms and figure. She says she threw out all her "fat" clothes.

Angel W., who had high blood pressure when she was 65 pounds

Keeping a Success Diary

How can teens who are just starting their journey to a healthier weight focus on the payback when they're not even there yet? One way to begin the process is to keep a "success diary," starting on day one of a weight journey, the way David G. did when he kept track of how he was doing on his calendar. The diary might include daily achievements—no matter how small—so teens learn to focus on their successes, which should bolster their motivation. The diary also might include small changes—in body, mind, and spirit—that take place on the way to a healthier weight. This should jump-start the process of recognizing the payback from developing a healthier lifestyle, even if teens aren't yet where they ultimately want to be.

For example, the success diary of a teen who has lost 15 of the 50 pounds she's trying to lose might look like this.

Today's successes:

- Got up early enough to have a bowl of oatmeal and a banana before school.
- Had a grilled chicken sandwich and diet soda instead of a burger, shake, and fries when we went to Burger King after school.
- Took stairs instead of the escalator at the mall.
- Walked the dog for thirty minutes after dinner.
- When angry at my mom, called a friend instead of raiding the fridge.

Changes in me:

- Have more energy.
- Feel better about myself.
- Jeans are getting looser.
- Can walk farther without getting out of breath.

When teens feel discouraged or have setbacks, they can pull out the success diary to remind themselves of the many positive changes that have already taken place.

heavier, stays motivated by knowing that she'd have health problems if she gained the weight back. Mike D. says, "I need to stay in shape because I do a lot of activities, so I can't be tired." Summer A. hopes to get a volleyball scholarship to college and stays motivated by thinking, "Is it worth gaining weight and not getting a scholarship?"

A number of teens stay motivated by both recalling the past *and* thinking about the payback. Tom C. looks at old photos and recalls how people made fun of him. But he also thinks about "how good I look in clothes, how good I feel, and how much better other kids treat me."

LIFE ONLY GETS BETTER

I asked the teens to evaluate how weight loss has affected the following areas of their lives using a rating scale. The responses from 92 of the teens show the payback from their efforts.

- Improved self-esteem and confidence: 99%.
- Improved level of energy: 90%.
- Improved moods and level of happiness: 87%.
- Improved physical health: 96%.
- Improved interactions with friends and peers: 84%.

For all of the aspects of life listed above, not one teen said that things had worsened or even "somewhat worsened." (A small number said there was "no difference.")

I also asked the teens how they feel about their body image, and 9 out of 10 indicated improvement. Eight said "no difference," and just one said "somewhat worsened."

Finally, when asked to rate time spent thinking about food (improvement meaning they think about it less), more than half of the teens said this had improved; about a third of them said "no difference;" 8 said "somewhat worsened"; and one said "greatly worsened." Given the vigilance required to maintain weight loss—particularly in a society that sets people up to eat too much and exercise too little—it's not surprising that some teens think about food more now than before. What *is* surprising is that so many of them think about food less or no more than when they were heavy.

These findings should be reassuring to people who are concerned that even sensible weight loss will lead most overweight teens to obsess about food and their bodies. David G. says, "I don't think about food nearly as much as I did before losing weight. Granted, I still have a passion for food and cooking, but it's not the same. When I was heavier, I couldn't wait to eat. And during unsuccessful diets, I would always be focused on the foods that I couldn't have. It was only when I learned that I could still eat basically any food I wanted — as long as it was in moderation — that I stopped thinking about food so much."

It Gets Easier

As David G.'s story illustrates, maintaining a healthy weight takes vigilance. I asked the teens the extent to which they agree with the statement "As time goes on, it gets easier to keep my weight down," using a rating scale. Of the 94 young people who answered the question, more than half agreed, about 20 percent were neutral, and about 20 percent disagreed.

I also asked the teens, "How hard is it to stay at your new weight?" More than half indicated that it's easy for them, just over a third chose neutral ground, and seven teens indicated that it's difficult.

Three quarters of the teens who've been successfully managing their weight for two or more years indicated that it's getting easier with time, while less than a third of the teens who've been at it for less than two years said this. Findings from the National Weight Control Registry also suggest that the longer formerly overweight people can keep extra pounds off, the easier it becomes.

None of this is to say that losing or maintaining weight is easy, and there's no question that it's harder for some teens than for others. My findings suggest that the teens who lost weight with the help of a program or a professional were *less likely* to say that maintaining their weight loss has gotten easier with time and *more likely* to say that it's been difficult to maintain the loss than were those who lost weight on their own. One explanation for this difference might be that the teens who needed help with their weight loss had a weight problem that was, for some reason, more intractable than that of the teens who lost weight on their own.

Joe M., who lost 60 pounds more than a decade ago (he also grew five inches) with the help of the medically supervised program Health Management Resources, says, "Losing weight has to be one of the most difficult things I've done in my life. It takes a lot of determination, and that must come from inside. Once I had the determination, then it required more work and change than I'd ever expected. You need to work hard at eating less and exercising more. Honestly, though, it's so great once you get going. After you get past the hard part, it actually gets easier, and life becomes much better."

A Permanent Change in Mindset

When I asked David G. about his "change in mindset," he responded, "I don't just tell myself, 'I've got to go work out.' Instead, I see things more as 'I get to do this' and 'It's going to be fun.'"

Julie Germann, Ph.D., clinical director of the FitMatters teen weight program at La Rabida Children's Hospital in Chicago, has observed this shift in mindset in successful participants. She says, "They find something enjoyable about what they're doing. For example, one girl who enjoys doodling in her journal has not missed a day of writing down what she eats and how much she exercises in the one and one half years she's been in our program. Another girl became successful after finding a very active sport she loved, so it doesn't feel so much like exercise."

Another critical shift in thinking that the teens expressed is that they moved away from a "dieting" mentality to one of accepting the need to make permanent changes that they can live with for the rest of their lives. David G. says, "One of the most important things I do to keep the weight off is that I continue to do what helped me lose the weight."

Emily B. puts it another way: "Weight loss is not just something you do, but a way of life. In order to keep the weight off, you have to acquire better eating habits during the process of losing weight."

Rebecca M. says, "I think the difference between a 'diet' and a lifestyle is that people who are on diets see it as only a temporary thing. Someone on a diet might say, 'Once I lose my weight, I can go back to eating good food or the way I used to eat again.' But a lifestyle is a permanent thing. I choose to eat the way I do and exercise because I never want to look the way I used to. I've found foods that are healthy *and* good to eat, so I don't feel like I'm just eating this way temporarily, until I go back to the way I used to eat."

Some teens don't even feel they need to "stay motivated" anymore because the changes they've made have become part of them. My son Wes says, "By making a total lifestyle change, I took away the need for motivation. This is just how I live now." Similarly, Mick J. says, "The way I see it, I've made a change in my life, as opposed to going on a diet. So I never have the sense that I need to keep anything off."

It's All About Choices

As Amber M. points out, successful weight management is all about making choices. She says, "My motivation to lose 152 pounds is still not clear, and it's been twelve years since I started the journey. But I think it all starts with a choice to be something different or take a different path than the one you're currently traveling. Something makes you think, 'Wow, I deserve so much more than this' and 'I can do anything I want.' Once this aha moment arrives, the remaining journey continues to be filled with choices. You have a choice each day about whether to exercise, eat properly, take care of yourself mentally — or to accept that there are going to be setbacks. You have a choice each day to better yourself."

Aaron T. concludes, "Once you see what it's like, you never, ever want to go back."

Weight Programs
Used by the Teens

Much of the information about the following weight management programs was provided by the programs themselves.* For the most current details about their approaches, costs, training of personnel, and studies on their effectiveness, contact each program directly. Families should proceed cautiously and thoughtfully when considering any weight program. See the guidelines in chapter 4 for evaluating weight programs.

Careful consideration should be given to the credentials and training of the people who deliver program content, as well as to the adequacy of the diet and whether it's designed to meet the needs of adolescents. Teens and their parents should check with their physicians about the appropriateness of any program or dietary approach for their individual needs. Consulting a registered dietitian may be helpful as well.

As Karen Miller-Kovach, M.S., R.D., points out in the book *Weight Watchers Family Power,* popular adult-based weight programs have not been adapted for or carefully studied in children and teens. To my knowledge, many of the well-known kids' weight programs have not been rigorously studied either. However, to varying degrees, these children's programs incorporate many of the strategies suggested to be effective for weight management in scientific studies involving young people.

---

* Inclusion of a program does not signify endorsement. A few of these programs offer supplements that have not been shown to be safe and effective for weight loss, particularly in teens. In some programs, employees receive a commission for signing up new members and/or selling products.

NATIONAL PROGRAMS

Adult-Oriented Programs

Curves

Program overview and philosophy: Curves is a fitness center franchise program designed to provide "a fast, fun, and efficient workout in a comfortable environment" where "women support and encourage each other." Most of its members are women who were previously not exercising. Curves offers a thirty-minute workout designed to provide strength training and cardiovascular activity at the same time. Although Curves franchises are primarily viewed as exercise facilities, they've recently made "a huge commitment to become a one-stop exercise and weight loss center," with increasing emphasis on a weight management program, which includes a choice of diets. The diets are encouraged in combination with exercise if members have more than 20 pounds to lose "and need the extra help." Members can follow the diets on their own or join the six-week Solution classes offered periodically at some Curves franchises. Behavior modification/motivational materials are available in written and CD format. Curves also offers a line of herbal and nutrition products.

Ages of clients served: Curves members are primarily adults age thirty-five and up, but many facilities allow young girls to join. It's up to each club to set an age minimum—for most it's ten to thirteen years of age. Young people follow the same program and use the same materials as adults. However, children under the age of eighteen must be signed up by a parent or added to a parent's membership. Parents do not have to accompany children and teens to workouts. Curves is currently testing its exercise program and a nutrition curriculum at several middle schools. (Curves will have new equipment in the near future and plans to donate its old equipment to middle schools.)

How participant progress is measured: During the first visit to Curves, a "figure analysis" is done that includes an interview about the person's health, current lifestyle, weight, body measurements, and personal goals. According to Curves headquarters, "Working together, the member and the trainer agree on an appropriate and attainable goal." Members are weighed and measured monthly, and a body fat analysis is done with a handheld device.

Dietary approach(es): Although many people use Curves solely for its exercise program, Curves also has its own weight management program. It offers a Higher Protein Diet or a Higher Carbohydrate Diet—both of which consist of three phases, starting out with about 1,200 calories per day for the first week, then increasing to 1,600 calories for the second phase. (Curves uses its own written "tests" for "carbohydrate intolerance" and to determine which diet participants should follow.) The third phase is not considered "dieting" and consists of 2,000 to 2,600 calories most of the time—with a 1,200-calorie diet to be used intermittently if the person gains three pounds. There is no special dietary approach for children and teens. Curves allows them to follow its diets and attend weight classes without a physician's recommendation.

Approaches for increasing physical activity: Curves uses a circuit system with a series of eight to twelve machines. Participants do as many repetitions as they can in thirty seconds on each machine. "Recovery stations," located between machines, are available for doing just about anything—from dancing to stretching to jogging—as long as you keep moving. Prerecorded lively music is designed to make the workout fun. Members are encouraged to do the Curves workout three times a week, adding other exercise in between workouts if they choose. Each workout includes "warmup, strength training, cardiovascular exercise, cooldown, and stretching."

Staff training and background: Curves franchise owners are required to take part in a weeklong company training geared primarily toward business operations. The Curves workout program is supervised by the Curves instructor on duty. These same instructors can teach Solution classes after they take part in a three- to four-hour training session. Instructors generally are not professionals and are often people who have benefited from the program. Cardiopulmonary resuscitation (CPR) certification is required for each employee. With the Cooper Institute, Curves recently set up its own certification program for people who work at Curves. This entails going through the weeklong company training and taking two college-level courses—one in general nutrition and another one in kinesiology, anatomy, physiology, or a similar field of study. The Curves program was designed with input from a licensed psychologist, a medical doctor, a registered dietitian, and exercise experts.

Published studies on program: Curves has funded a multimillion-dollar research initiative at Baylor University to study the program's efficacy. A number of studies have been presented at scientific meetings, and a few of them have been published in scientific journals.

Program costs: The fee to join Curves is $149, but special deals are sometimes offered. Additional fees run about $29 to $49 per month, depending on the location. The Solution classes cost extra.

Maintenance program/program follow-up: There is no separate maintenance program. Members are encouraged to continue coming to Curves indefinitely.

Geographic locations: Curves has franchises in fifty states and thirty-eight foreign countries, with more than 7,800 locations in the United States.

Phone: (800) 848-1096

Web site: www.curves.com

Health Management Resources (HMR)

Program overview and philosophy: HMR describes itself as follows: "The HMR Program is a problem-solving, educational approach that teaches skills for long-term weight and health management. With a commitment to developing healthy lifestyles, the focus is on increasing physical activity, increasing vegetable and fruit intake, and using nutritious shakes, entrées, and bars [meal replacements] in place of all or some meals to lower dietary fat and calorie intake." HMR uses a weekly group format and a midweek phone check-in with a staff member, or "coach." Members receive practical, hands-on training through the use of assignments and evaluation of their own food and exercise records. The program incorporates behavioral strategies for lifestyle modification.

Ages of clients served: Although the HMR program was designed for adults, many adolescents have been treated in its program. The program accepts girls between the ages of twelve and eighteen and boys between thirteen and eighteen — after a physician has screened them to verify that they have completed most of their growth. Currently, younger children are not treated in the program. Parents or guardians of teens are encouraged to accompany them to the weekly group meetings as a way to learn the program basics. Although HMR does not have a separate program for teens at this time, some locations may offer teen groups. (HMR is in the process of developing an adolescent program that allows teens to participate in phone-based follow-up for both weight loss and maintenance.)

How participant progress is measured: The overall focus of the HMR approach is on health, not just weight. As such, a weight goal is not established. Weekly progress is measured not only by weight loss but also by compliance with the diet, physical activity goals, and vegetable and fruit intake goals.

Dietary approach(es): Meal replacements are used in all the diet plans as a way to provide structure and reduce calorie intake, but HMR offers a choice of several diet options. The more intensive one is physician directed, uses only meal replacements, and provides a minimum of 1,000 calories per day. Another plan combines meal replacements with five 1-cup servings of vegetables and fruits and ranges from 1,275 to 1,475 calories per day. Both plans meet the nutritional needs of teens who fit the program criteria.

Approaches for increasing physical activity: Participants are taught how to track and calculate physical activity calories. Calories are estimated based on level of intensity and duration of activity. The goal is a minimum of 2,000 calories of physical activity per week.

Staff training and background: The HMR program is delivered by a multidisciplinary team, including physicians, nurses, registered dietitians, and trained health educators. All staff members participate in intensive initial and ongoing training. The HMR program was developed by health care professionals, including physicians, nurses, dietitians, and behavioral psychologists.

Published studies on program: HMR has published a number of studies on its approach and regularly presents data at professional conferences.

Program costs: The cost of the HMR program varies depending on the level of medical supervision required and meal replacement product charges. In general, the one-time induction fee ranges from $63 to $241 (including a clinical evaluation, laboratory tests, a health risk appraisal, educational materials, a physical exam when required, and an introductory behavioral group). Subsequent fees average $20 to $50 per week for lifestyle education and medical supervision, if required. Weekly meal replacement purchases range from $66 to $87 and replace the usual costs of grocery store food. Health insurance reimbursement depends on individual plans and medical diagnosis.

Maintenance program/program follow-up: HMR is known for its commitment to maintenance and its long-term program. The maintenance program provides an opportunity for continued practice in the same lifestyle behaviors learned during weight loss. The cost of maintenance averages $20 per week. Some participants prefer the option of participating in a phone-based program for maintenance.

Geographic locations: HMR programs are located nationwide. There are approximately 150 programs in 35 states.

Phone: (800) 418-1367

Web site: www.hmrprogram.com

Jenny Craig

Program overview and philosophy: Jenny Craig uses "a comprehensive food/body/mind approach to long-term weight management by helping clients create a healthy relationship with food, build an active lifestyle, and develop a balanced approach to living." The program is offered at centers that clients go to weekly for one-on-one counseling that addresses balanced nutrition, portion control, physical activity, and motivation. Participants purchase varying amounts of preportioned Jenny Craig food products, depending on which food plan they follow. Jenny Craig incorporates cognitive-behavioral strategies, including realistic goal setting, tracking of food intake and activity, controlling environmental cues that promote unplanned eating, problem solving, dealing with emotional eating, and cognitive restructuring.

Ages of clients served: Though primarily designed for adults, Jenny Craig will accept teens age thirteen and up—with their parents' written permission—provided they do not have preexisting health conditions, are not on medication, and are not pregnant or breastfeeding. According to the company, "The greater goal of the Jenny Craig Adolescent Program is to help participants develop healthy attitudes and behaviors around food and physical activity versus lose a specific amount of weight." When teens enroll in the program, a Jenny Craig consultant meets with them once a week. The teens' parents are also given program materials that reinforce the key role they play in their children's success. Many teen clients have parents who are also in the Jenny Craig program.

How participant progress is measured: Clients choose a realistic weight goal based on healthy weight ranges for adolescents, as well as factors such as personal and family weight history and level of motivation. Progress is measured by weekly weigh-ins, monthly body measurements, and monthly assessment of food/body/mind behavioral changes on a "lifestyle graph." For teens, the program is designed so they can lose one half to one pound per week, "in order to support calorie needs for growth." However, teens may choose to maintain their current weight, with a goal of growing into it over time. (For adults, menus are designed to result in a loss of one to two pounds or 1 percent of current weight per week.)

Dietary approach(es): Jenny Craig offers clients weekly menu

plans featuring varying levels of Jenny Craig breakfast, lunch, and dinner entrées and snacks — depending on the client's lifestyle, phase of
weight loss, and personal preferences. Menus are complemented by the
client's own fruits and vegetables, nonfat milk/yogurt, and other foods.
Adolescent females receive a 1,500-calorie menu unless they have more
than 80 pounds to lose, in which case they receive a 1,700-calorie
menu. Boys receive a 1,700-calorie menu unless they have more than 80
pounds to lose, in which case they receive a 2,000-calorie menu. The
overall emphasis is on lowering fat intake and eating more fruits, vegetables, and whole grains, particularly as clients switch over to preparing more of their own foods when approaching their goal weight. Participants also receive a multivitamin/mineral supplement.

Approaches for increasing physical activity: Jenny Craig's physical
activity component was developed in consultation with the Cooper Institute, which uses research-based strategies matched to individuals'
level of motivation and personalized to their preferences and lifestyle.
Clients receive information about this at weekly visits and are expected
to follow through at home. Jenny Craig also offers exercise audiotapes
and videotapes geared toward beginning, intermediate, and advanced
fitness levels. Parents are encouraged to plan physically active family
time together to support their teen's efforts.

Staff training and background: The Jenny Craig consultants who
meet with clients weekly receive forty hours of training on the basics of
nutrition, exercise, and behavioral change for weight management.
They attend an additional training course to receive a certificate in "active lifestyle facilitation skills" from the Cooper Institute. All employees
also attend monthly continuing education classes delivered by field
trainers. The ongoing development of the Jenny Craig program involves
licensed psychologists, registered dietitians, medical doctors, exercise
physiologists, and respected experts working in the field of behavior
change and weight management.

Published studies on program: Jenny Craig has not published studies on its approach in scientific journals, but it has presented them at professional meetings. The company is in the process of doing a study to evaluate its effectiveness, and the Cooper Institute has done an independent analysis of clients' weight loss success rates.

Program costs: The cost to enroll in Jenny Craig's adolescent program is $98 for twelve months. If a teen still has weight to lose after one year, he or she may purchase another twelve-month program for $98. The cost of the more than seventy-five prepackaged Jenny's Cuisine food items is $11 to $15 per day in the United States. Jenny Craig has an arrangement with some health insurance companies that cover, discount, or reimburse subscribers for some of the costs.

Maintenance program/program follow-up: Although Jenny Craig offers adults a maintenance program for an additional cost, it does not have a separate maintenance program for teens.

Geographic locations: Jenny Craig has approximately six hundred centers in the United States, Canada, Australia, New Zealand, Puerto Rico, and Guam.

Phone: (800) 597-JENNY

Web site: www.jennycraig.com

L A Weight Loss Centers

Program overview and philosophy: L A Weight Loss Centers provide customized meal plans and a balanced diet—using your own foods, not prepackaged ones—as well as one-on-one weight loss counseling with company-trained counselors. Centers are either company owned or franchised. L A Weight Loss offers a three-phase program. During the first, or weight loss, phase, counselors meet with clients three times a week to discuss challenges, provide advice and strategies for adhering to the diet, and offer encouragement and support. (See "maintenance program/program follow-up" for information on the other two phases.) According to the company, its program focus is "nutritional counseling and teaching clients to make smart food decisions and limit portion sizes, while unlearning their bad food habits developed over their life-time." The program also offers its own line of nutrition supplements and "weight loss enhancers," which include nutrition bars and herbal supplements. (According to the company, "teens may not be eligible for the weight loss enhancers.")

Ages of clients served: The typical age of participants is twenty-five to fifty-five, but L A Weight Loss accepts children over the age of six if their primary care physician signs a form that allows the young person to join the program. Teens are generally eligible for the program, and there's a specific meal plan for them. Parents are encouraged to attend weekly meetings with their children. According to the company, "program counselors work with the parents and the family physician to en-sure that adolescent participants receive the proper weight loss counsel-ing."

How participant progress is measured: A healthy goal weight is de-termined for each participant with the help of her or his weight loss counselor. The goal is one with which clients feel comfortable, not a weight determined according to charts. Progress is measured through weekly weigh-ins, monthly body measurements, and a review of eating habits as noted in each client's food diary. The company guarantees weight loss of two pounds per week.

Dietary approach(es): The L A Weight Loss program's personalized menu plans for teenagers are designed by a team of registered dietitians to meet teens' nutritional needs and provide between 1,700 and 2,100 calories per day. Counselors encourage teens to eat a variety of foods for a balanced diet and to monitor their portion sizes while making room for "fun foods" in moderation.

Approaches for increasing physical activity: L A Weight Loss "strongly encourages clients to get active." The program offers tapes that help inactive people begin an exercise program.

Staff training and background: Many of the counselors are former or existing clients of L A Weight Loss. They take part in a six-week company training on all aspects of the program, "from nutrition, to our products, to how to help clients overcome common diet obstacles." The L A Weight Loss diet and meal plans are "continually evaluated and upgraded by the company's numerous staff dietitians," who are available to counselors as needed. The program has a physician consultant who acts as medical director.

Published studies on program: L A Weight Loss has not published studies on its approach in scientific journals. However, it conducts "internal studies" on an ongoing basis that focus on average weight loss and program compliance "in an effort to improve the program."

Program costs: Costs of the program vary by location, by franchise, and by the amount of weight you want to lose. Clients pay for the program up front. On average, costs run about $8 a week for all phases of the program. Health insurance coverage varies.

Maintenance program/program follow-up: After clients meet their goal weight, they go through a six-week stabilization phase in which foods are added to the diet. During this phase, clients meet with their counselors twice a week. Following stabilization is the maintenance phase—a yearlong period in which clients meet with a counselor just once a week.

Geographic locations: Worldwide, there are about 750 L A Weight Loss Centers, 650 of which are located throughout the forty-eight contiguous states.

Phone: (800) 526-SLIM or (800) 331-4035

Web site: www.laweightloss.com

Take Off Pounds Sensibly (TOPS)

Program overview and philosophy: TOPS is a nonprofit, noncommercial organization consisting of a network of "associate chapters" that provide group support for weight loss. People may join an existing chapter or start their own with a minimum of four members. An international headquarters offers members healthy food plans, educational materials, and other tools for weight loss. According to headquarters, "TOPS offers fellowship as people change to a healthier, new lifestyle and learn to maintain it." Chapter members meet weekly to weigh in and discuss diet and exercise methods, using professionally prepared programs. Other topics covered may include meal planning, motivation, goal setting, challenges, and emotional aspects of eating. Each chapter is unique and run by its members, who choose how topics will be addressed.

Ages of clients served: TOPS chapters primarily include adults but accept children as young as age seven. Children and teens often join with a parent or guardian, but this is not required. Adults may start chapters specifically for children.

How participant progress is measured: TOPS members may select their own weight goal, although TOPS recommends that they seek guidance from a health care professional. Progress is recorded each week at the member's weigh-in. Weight loss is recognized with a local, regional, and national reward system and in competitions based on improvement and/ or number of pounds lost. Special divisions exist for children and teens.

Dietary approach(es): Since TOPS's mission is to support people during weight loss and maintenance and to make tools available for managing the process, it does not advocate a particular dietary approach or sell a food program. Its philosophy is that members must find a weight loss method that's right for them. The organization does offer a guidebook that provides a food "exchange system" of varying calorie levels and outlines how to use the food pyramid to create a healthy food plan. TOPS recommends that members consult a health care professional for nutritional guidance, but this is not required.

Approaches for increasing physical activity: Members are encouraged to incorporate exercise into their lives, under the guidance of a health care professional. Exercise/movement tips are included in weekly programs. The TOPS lifestyle guide, *The Choice Is Mine,* features a section on aerobics, walking, and strength and flexibility exercises.

Staff training and background: Weekly meetings are run by volunteer leaders, but weekly programs can be presented by any member.

Leaders are not required to have formal training, but they do receive professionally prepared educational materials on weight management and health from TOPS headquarters. TOPS chapters are overseen by a field staff that helps them operate. TOPS materials are designed with involvement from a medical doctor, licensed psychologist, and registered dietitian.

Published studies on program: TOPS has not published studies on its approach in scientific journals. Each year, the organization publishes *Fabulous Figures*, a comprehensive report that outlines membership weight gains and losses.

Program costs: The fee for joining TOPS is $24 in the United States and $30 in Canada. Children and teens receive a reduced rate. Each chapter sets its own dues, which typically run from $2 to $5 per month.

Maintenance program/program follow-up: TOPS members who are keeping off pounds (maintainers, called KOPS, for Keep Off Pounds Sensibly) are encouraged to remain in their chapters because TOPS believes that support is needed at every stage of weight management — beginners and maintainers help each other. According to headquarters, "TOPS views weight loss as part of lifestyle management, not a certain period of time." Generally speaking, there are not separate meetings for maintainers. A section of *The Choice Is Mine* is devoted to maintenance and includes recommendations from the National Weight Control Registry.

Geographic locations: TOPS has 200,000 members in 9,000 chapters in every state and province throughout the United States and Canada. It has 100 chapters overseas.

Phone: (800) 932-8677

Web site: www.tops.org

Weight Watchers

Program overview and philosophy: According to the company, "Weight Watchers provides a comprehensive weight management program built on four pillars — healthful reduced-calorie food plans, regular physical activity, a supportive atmosphere, and constructive thinking/behavior skills." The program offers Tools for Living, which include strategies such as problem-solving and coping skills. Weight Watchers has a group format with weekly meetings.

Ages of clients served: Although Weight Watchers does not encourage children to join its program, it accepts young people ages ten through seventeen with a physician's referral. (Anyone who has been diagnosed with an eating disorder or who is pregnant is not allowed to join.) Since Weight Watchers does not currently have a specific program geared toward adolescents, it's up to the parents of kids in the program to determine the extent to which they want to be involved. Weight Watchers is in the process of developing a family-based program designed to create a "healthy weight" home environment for kids and adults alike. Information about this program can be found at www.weightwatchers.com/family.

How participant progress is measured: Weekly weigh-ins are part of the program. For members under the age of eighteen, Weight Watchers requires that a weight goal be established by the child's physician. For those eighteen and older, the initial recommended weight loss goal is 10 percent of starting weight. The final goal is to achieve a healthy weight — a BMI between 20 and 25 or a weight deemed healthy for that individual by a health care professional.

Dietary approach(es): Weight Watchers' members can choose from two different dietary approaches. The Flex Plan or POINTS Food System uses a counting method in which foods are assigned a POINTS value and participants are allotted a daily POINTS target to "spend" as they choose. The newer Core Plan (described as a "no counting system") is more structured and uses a list of nutritious foods that are relatively low in calories and have low "abuse potential." According to Weight Watchers, following either plan should result in a weight loss of one to two pounds per week. Both plans have a weekly allowance for "treats" to prevent feelings of deprivation.

Approaches for increasing physical activity: Weight Watchers'

POINTS Activity System provides a method to measure and track exercise. It's based on body weight, time spent in the activity, and the intensity at which the activity is performed. The system begins with reducing sedentary behavior, then gradually increases the role of physical activity so that by the time a person has reached his or her ultimate weight goal, he or she is doing 60 to 90 minutes of moderate activity each day.

Staff training and background: Weekly meetings are facilitated by company-trained members who have been through the program, completed a three- to four-day training, and are maintaining a healthy body weight. Ongoing training and regular coaching are also provided several times each year. The Weight Watchers program is designed by a team of health care professionals, including registered dietitians, physicians, exercise physiologists, and clinical psychologists.

Published studies on program: Weight Watchers has published several studies involving adults in scientific journals, comparing its approach to other weight loss approaches.

Program costs: The program charges a registration fee of about $15 (often waived as part of a promotion) and a weekly meeting fee of $12 to $14. Several insurance plans provide some coverage for Weight Watchers.

Maintenance program/program follow-up: Once members reach their goal weight, they are encouraged to continue to attend weekly meetings for six weeks. This is considered the maintenance phase. (There are no separate meetings for maintainers.) Beyond that time, attendance at a meeting on at least a monthly basis is recommended. As an incentive to participate in an ongoing fashion, those who become "lifetime members" (that is, complete the weight loss and maintenance phases of the program) attend meetings at no charge as long as they are within two pounds of their goal weight.

Geographic locations: Weight Watchers conducts approximately 46,000 weekly meetings in 30 countries around the world.

Phone: (800) 651-6000

Web site: www.weightwatchers.com

Programs Designed for Youth

SHAPEDOWN

Program overview and philosophy: SHAPEDOWN is a family-based behavior modification and skill development program developed for children and adolescents. The program is usually delivered once a week over a ten-week period—in either a group or individual counseling format—by a health care professional. It begins with an individualized assessment to define the underlying causes of and contributors to each child's weight or eating problems, then devises strategies to address those problems. SHAPEDOWN puts a strong emphasis on physical activity, dealing with emotional eating, problem solving, cognitive restructuring, limit setting, family communication, building self-esteem, and parenting skills.

Ages of clients served: SHAPEDOWN offers two programs, one for children ages six to twelve and another for adolescents ages twelve to twenty. Both programs require parental attendance at all sessions, and parents must be involved in the behavior change assignments to be done at home. SHAPEDOWN transfers more responsibility from the parent to the child in the teen program.

How participant progress is measured: Kids are weighed once a week by the program provider. The goal is steady weight loss, at a suggested rate of one pound per week. (SHAPEDOWN does not allow weight loss of more than two pounds per week.) In addition, SHAPEDOWN offers providers a range of assessment/evaluation instruments, such as the Family Habit Inventory, a fitness profile, and a more detailed profile of the family and the child's weight, knowledge, and behavior. This computerized assessment instrument identifies issues that contribute to weight or eating problems. Follow-up assessments are used to monitor participants' progress toward goals.

Dietary approach(es): SHAPEDOWN uses no specific diet. "Rather, education is provided about nutrition, caloric density, the food pyramid, label reading, and the consequences of various food choices." "Free," "light," "heavy," and "junk" food categories are defined. Families are taught how to determine caloric intake and are educated about the health risks involved in reducing daily intake to below 1,200 calories per day.

Approaches for increasing physical activity: Aerobic exercise is encouraged, individualized exercise goals are established, and progress toward goals is measured. Exercise takes place outside the program sessions. Parents are encouraged to exercise with their children.

Staff training and background: The SHAPEDOWN program is sold only to licensed and/or credentialed health care providers, such as medical doctors, registered nurses, registered dietitians, social workers, psychologists, and registered physical therapists. Would-be providers of the program must complete a forty-six-hour video course and pass an assessment before being certified and licensed as a SHAPEDOWN provider. The program was developed and is continuously updated by an interdisciplinary team at the University of California, San Francisco, School of Medicine. The team includes a medical doctor, licensed psychologist, registered dietitian, nurse practitioner, and exercise physiologist.

Published studies on program: In 1987, a study on SHAPEDOWN that involved adolescents was published in the *Journal of the American Dietetic Association.*

Program costs: SHAPEDOWN providers set their own prices, which vary widely. The national average for a ten-week group program is $375 to $400. The average cost when the program is used for individual counseling (one family at a time) is about $60 per hour. Some health insurance plans pay for at least part of the fees, particularly if the child has a weight-related medical condition.

Maintenance program/program follow-up: An optional ADVANCED SHAPEDOWN twenty-week maintenance program is available and may be repeated indefinitely. SHAPEDOWN's director estimates that the average weekly follow-up session costs about $30 per family.

210 WEIGHT LOSS CONFIDENTIAL

Geographic locations: SHAPEDOWN has more than nine hundred providers in the United States, as well as about two dozen in Europe, the Far East, and the Pacific Rim.

Phone: (415) 453-8886

Web site: www.shapedown.com

Trim Kids (formerly known as Committed to Kids or CTK)

Program overview and philosophy: Trim Kids was designed by a team of experts at the Louisiana State University (LSU) Health Sciences Center as an outpatient program to be conducted in a group setting over the course of twelve months. The program has been adapted for use in county programs, schools, YMCAs, health and fitness facilities, and private health practitioner offices. (Many of the Trim Kids affiliate programs are three to six months in duration and do not have all of the components described here. The description here applies to the model program, as it exists at LSU. When considering other Trim Kids programs, check with the director to find out what they include.) The Trim Kids model is meant to be run by a team of professionals and is individualized according to each child's age, gender, medical history, degree of overweight, and fitness level. The program focuses on education about and application of healthy exercise, nutrition, and behavior modification strategies. Participants and their parents come to the program once a week for family-based group sessions.

Ages of clients served: Trim Kids is designed for kids ages five to seventeen, but it considers itself a family program. Parent participation is required. In fact, all family members are encouraged to come to sessions. Many sessions or parts of sessions are held with everyone together, while others are held with young people in one room and parents in another. Parents-only meetings address positive approaches to parenting. Children-only sessions focus on topics such as dealing with teasing and peer pressure. Some Trim Kids affiliates separate younger children from teens, but most combine these age groups.

How participant progress is measured: Short-term and long-term goals for weight, behavioral changes, exercise, and nutrition are established with input from the participants, parents, and health care professionals. Typically, participants are weighed weekly. In addition, at the outset, kids receive a comprehensive physical exam, blood tests, psychological tests, and exercise and nutrition evaluations. Over time, changes in these areas are evaluated so participants can see improvements in their health and physical fitness. Progress also is assessed with weekly goals and detailed food and activity records that participants are asked to keep.

Dietary approach(es): In the headquarters program, several different dietary approaches are employed. Children and teens who are "at the high end of the moderate range of overweight and in the severe range of overweight" are offered a very low-calorie diet called the protein-modified fast. This diet is a high-protein, low-carbohydrate diet of 900 to 1,100 calories per day and may be used only under a physician's supervision. Kids who are less overweight are offered a balanced reduced-calorie diet, which ranges from 1,200 to 2,400 calories a day, depending on age, gender, and government recommendations for young people. Most Trim Kids affiliate programs place participants on the balanced reduced-calorie regimen. Participants are asked to write down what they eat and to monitor their daily calorie intake in a food journal.

Approaches for increasing physical activity: The Trim Kids philosophy for physical activity is "Make it fun, and make it doable—and make sure the parents and interventionists are there doing the same thing alongside the youngsters!" The program is designed to include exercise at weekly meetings as well as at home. The program combines aerobic, strength, and flexibility exercises, which increase progressively as kids go through the program. Participants and their families are encouraged to reduce sedentary activities and to become more physically active outside the weekly sessions. Each week, achievable goals are set for kids to engage in a variety of activities, such as dancing, walking, bike riding, and playing sports and games. Participants are asked to keep track of their daily activities in a journal.

Staff training and background: The Trim Kids developers recommend that affiliates use a team approach that includes medical monitoring by a physician, nutrition education provided by a registered dietitian, exercise intervention by an exercise physiologist (or an individual certified in pediatric exercise or physical education), and behavior modification intervention by a child psychologist or other mental health professional. (A team of health care professionals like these developed the Trim Kids program.) However, some Trim Kids affiliates do not employ this level or variety of professionals. To set up an affiliate Trim Kids program, professionals should purchase mail-order materials detailed at the program Web site. Training with a Trim Kids developer is optional at an additional cost. No licensing, screening of purchasers, or franchising fees are required to set up a Trim Kids program.

Published studies on program: The Trim Kids developers have published many studies on various aspects of the program in scientific journals and presented their findings at numerous scientific meetings.

Program costs: The cost for a year of treatment at the headquarters Trim Kids program in New Orleans is $1,800 to $2,400. This includes all aspects of the program. Most health insurance companies cover the medical expenses, such as physical exams and lab work, and some cover consultation with other health care professionals. Some cover the program in its entirety. At affiliate sites, costs of the program vary widely, depending on the length of the program, the medical care and services provided, and the number of professionals involved. Some programs are "free" or county programs, and some are funded by grants.

Maintenance program/program follow-up: The Trim Kids headquarters program offers lifetime follow-up at no additional cost once a participant is enrolled and completes the recommended term of treatment, which varies from six months for children and teens who are less overweight to two years for those with severe obesity. The maintenance program is designed to reinforce a healthy family lifestyle by reviewing previously covered topics, as well as introducing new topics and community activities. Children and their families may attend weekly, monthly, or quarterly. However, the maintenance program varies from one Trim Kids affiliate to another, and most sites charge an additional fee for the maintenance program.

Geographic locations: Trim Kids programs can be found in more than a dozen states.

Phone number: Interested parties may contact one of the Trim Kids developers, T. Kristian von Almen, Ph.D., by e-mailing him at kvaphd@juno.com or call (408) 258-7062.

Web sites: www.trimkids.com. (A self-directed home version of the Trim Kids program, called *Trim Kids,* is available as a book for parents or health care professionals. The *Trim Kids* program is also available online through the Web site www.ediets.com.)

Way to Go Kids!

Program overview and philosophy: Way to Go Kids! was designed specifically for overweight children and teens by two dietitians, one of whom was overweight as a child. It's set up as an eight-week program that dietitians can purchase and run on their own. The program's primary goals are "to encourage lifestyle changes in kids and give them tools for lifelong success in weight management." The focus is on educating children and their parents about healthy eating and on increasing physical activity. Although the program was designed for group counseling, it can be used by dietitians who work with children on an individual basis. Group sessions are once a week for two hours: one hour is devoted to nutrition-related instruction and activities, and the other hour is for exercise. Classes also address behavior modification, body image, fitness activities, and emotional eating.

Ages of clients served: Way to Go Kids! targets children ages nine to twelve, and parents are strongly urged to accompany them to the classes.

The program includes three additional sessions for parents only. For teens, it's recommended that dietitians use the program outlines to provide individual counseling. The program developers also offer an adult program called FitWeigh, which may be used for older teens.

How participant progress is measured: No weight loss goals are established. The goals are to stop weight gain—while maintaining normal growth and development—and to change eating habits. According to the mission statement, however, "when kids get their portions under control and choose healthier options, there is often a weight loss." The child's weight status is discussed in the parents-only sessions.

Dietary approach(es): The main emphasis is on reducing fat and sugar intake, as well as understanding healthy portion sizes. The food pyramid is used as the basis for teaching about nutrition. Each week, kids participate in making and tasting simple, healthy recipes or reading labels to determine appropriate portion sizes. Calorie levels are not emphasized, although guidelines are given for healthy eating at a 1,600- to 1,800-calorie level. This is a guide, not a diet.

Approaches for increasing physical activity: One hour of each session is devoted to physical activity, such as playing dodge ball, jumping rope, taking a walk, exercising to music videotapes, or doing Tae Bo.

Staff training and background: It's recommended that a registered dietitian teach the nutrition component and that an exercise professional run the physical activity component. A registered dietitian must at least be available as a consultant. Dietitians are not required to have any training specific to the program, but support is available as needed from the program developers. The developers are both registered dietitians who have many years of experience with weight management, and one of them is a certified aerobics instructor. Both have special training in pediatric weight management provided by the American Dietetic Association.

Published studies on program: No published studies have been done on Way to Go Kids! However, data on the program are currently being analyzed with the assistance of a University of Alabama faculty member.

Program costs: It's up to the program provider to decide what to charge, but participants typically pay $100 to $300 for the program. It's difficult to receive insurance reimbursement for the program, although some coverage may be available.

Maintenance program/program follow-up: There is no separate maintenance program, mainly due to lack of interest.

Geographic locations: The program has been sold in more than 40 states, and more than 150 Way to Go Kids! programs are available in the United States.

Phone: (256) 880-6828

Web site: www.waytogokids.com

SMALLER PROGRAMS

Children's Weight Camps

Note: None of these camps has published studies on their program outcomes. Contact each camp directly for information about how it evaluates program effectiveness and about staff qualifications.

Camp La Jolla

Camp La Jolla is a residential summer fitness, weight loss, and health program located on the beach on the campus of the University of California, San Diego. (The camp is not affiliated with the university, however.) Campers range in age from eight to eighteen, with programs designed for each age group and gender. There's also a separate program for women ages eighteen to twenty-nine, a program for older women and mothers, and a one-week family camp. According to Nancy Lenhart, the camp's founder and director, "At Camp La Jolla, we believe that losing weight can be fun, safe, and long-term. We believe people are capable of achieving their goals when provided with personal choice, knowledge, and support from family, friends, and professionals." The program includes sports and other physical activities, as well as nutrition and behavior modification classes. The camp's mission is "to help people attain personal and fitness goals through noncompetitive, fun fitness activities, education, encouragement, and support." Each camper's weight and measurements are taken upon arrival, at two-week intervals, and upon departure. According to Ms. Lenhart, "Camp La Jolla follows the American Dietetic Association and American Heart Association guidelines for a healthy, well-balanced meal plan. We offer a minimum of 1,200 calories per day for females and 1,500 calories per day for males."

Camp La Jolla costs from $3,995 for a three-week stay to $9,195 for all nine weeks. Some scholarships are available. Campers are sent home with educational materials on nutrition and behavior modification and with fitness DVDs. Campers may take part in a two-year follow-up program, which includes a toll-free number for twenty-four-hour support, free conference calling between camper friends anywhere in the United States, monthly newsletters, fitness videos, and monthly weekend retreats. There's a fee for the retreats, but everything else listed as part of the follow-up program is free.

Phone: (800) 825-8746 or (800) 825-TRIM
Web site: www.camplajolla.com

Camp Shane

Camp Shane is a family-owned residential summer weight loss and fitness camp in the Catskill Mountains of New York. It offers campers many different sports, a pool and lake program, nutrition and cooking classes, rap sessions to help build self-esteem, arts and crafts, a theater program, and other recreational activities. Recently, a cognitive-behavioral therapy component was added. The program is coed for children ages eight to seventeen, and the camp offers a separate program for young women ages seventeen to twenty-five. One of the camp's goals is to help kids have fun while learning or improving athletic skills in a noncompetitive atmosphere. Although participants are weighed upon arrival, weekly, and at the end of the program, Camp Shane's spokesperson says, "We do not set specific weight loss goals. Our philosophy is to not dwell on weight loss, which will naturally occur with a healthier balance of fewer calories and more activity." Camp Shane's nutrition philosophy is based on "balanced, portion-controlled, kid-friendly food," but it tries to limit fat intake and sugar while serving lots of fruits and vegetables. The calorie level is about 1,600 per day.

Camp Shane has three-, six-, and nine-week sessions, at a cost of approximately $3,000, $5,000, and $7,000, respectively. The camp offers some limited scholarships. When kids return home, the camp makes an attempt to match campers and their families with a dietitian for follow-up care. Rebates are provided for families who follow through with this care or who arrange for their children to attend a weight program at home. Campers are also given a *Home Manual* and are sent monthly nutrition and fitness newsletters.

Phone: (845) 292-4644 (during the summer) or (914) 271-4141 (during the winter)

Web site: www.campshane.com

New Image Camps / Camp Pocono Trails

New Image Camps are residential summer weight loss camps located at three different sites — in Florida, California, and Pennsylvania. Camp Pocono Trails, located in Pennsylvania's Pocono Mountains, referred a number of teens for this book. Campers range in age from seven to eighteen. According to the director and owner, Tony Sparber, "The focus of the camps is on losing weight, gaining self-esteem, and having fun — all in a nonthreatening, stress-free environment." They offer many different noncompetitive sports, exercise classes, water activities, nutrition and cooking classes, arts and crafts, a class in charm and poise, a drama class, and other recreational activities. Campers also participate in self-esteem workshops and rap sessions to deal with the emotional aspects of eating. An important goal is to make fitness fun and to help campers find some type of physical activity that they enjoy and can continue when they return home. The calorie level of the food program is 1,700 to 2,000 per day, and campers are weighed once a week to monitor progress.

The camp costs approximately $1,000 per week, but this varies depending on how long the child stays. (Some campers have received outside funding from a private hospital, and single parents may receive a discount.) When campers go home, they're given a book designed to help them, and their parents, follow through with what they learned and did at camp. Parents and campers are also able to call during the year and speak with the camps' professionals if they have any questions or concerns. Mr. Sparber recently started a postcamp Internet counseling and support program that will be free for campers for a period of time after they return home. New Image also has some follow-up year-round afterschool programs in several states. (The afterschool programs and Internet programs are available to noncampers, too.)

Phone: (800) 365-0556

Web site: www.newimagecamp.com

Dietitians' Programs and One-of-a-Kind Programs

The following dietitians and smaller programs referred teens for this book. Contact them directly for costs and to find out how they evaluate their programs.

Back to Basics Nutrition Consulting

Back to Basics Nutrition Consulting is the private practice of nutrition consultant Lisa Bunce, M.S., R.D., located in West Redding, Connecticut. She offers "an individualized approach toward wellness" using behavioral/goal-oriented strategies. She works with children and adults of all ages.

Phone: (203) 938-0492
E-mail: lvbunce@optonline.net

Comprehensive Weight Management Center, Cincinnati Children's Hospital Medical Center

The center offers several different approaches for child and adolescent weight management, using an interdisciplinary team that includes physicians, registered dietitians, psychologists, exercise physiologists, and nurses. One program offered by the center is HealthWorks!, directed by registered dietitian Shelley Kirk, Ph.D., which uses individual nutrition counseling, group exercise sessions, behavior change strategies, and parent involvement. The center also has an obesity surgery program designed specifically for teens. The surgical director is Thomas Inge, M.D., Ph.D. (For more on the surgical option, see chapter 4.)

Phone: HealthWorks!: (513) 636-4305; surgical program: (800) 344-2462

Web site: www.cchmc.org/weight

FitMatters

A weight control program located at La Rabida Children's Hospital in Chicago, FitMatters was developed for children and teens ages eight to eighteen by psychologist Daniel Kirschenbaum, Ph.D., and its clinical director is another psychologist, Julie Germann, Ph.D. FitMatters is a comprehensive multidisciplinary program — also involving a registered dietitian, physical therapist, social worker, and physician — that targets family lifestyle change. The primary component of FitMatters is weekly cognitive-behavioral group therapy for children and their parents. (Parent participation is required.) Participants also attend monthly nutrition and exercise classes. The program encourages a very low-fat diet (less than 20 grams of fat per day) and a less structured goal of 1,200 to 1,400 calories per day. A major focus is the importance of accurate self-monitoring of fat, calorie, and activity levels. The program is open-ended, but participants are encouraged to commit to at least one year in order to achieve habit change.

Phone: (773) 256-5733

Web site: www.larabida.org

Healthy Directions

Healthy Directions is a group weight and lifestyle program designed to be run by a registered dietitian—ideally, with an exercise physiologist. According to the program creator, Mary Gilmore, R.D., "our goal is to take scientific information regarding diet and lifestyle and show individuals how to realistically apply it to their personal lives. Our program is unique in that it has no specific starting date or ending date; participants are encouraged to remain in the program as long as they feel they are benefiting and need support." Healthy Directions is primarily an adult program, but several children have attended with their parents. The program's lessons address topics such as healthful eating, exercise, relapse prevention, emotional eating, and stress management. Healthy Directions is available as a written or CD-ROM program that dietitians can purchase and run on their own. The program has been sold to more than one hundred registered dietitians, but Ms. Gilmore must be contacted directly for information about whether there's a program in a particular area.

Phone: (601) 482-2337

Web site: www.healthydirections.info

Marshfield Clinic Pediatrics Department

Located in Marshfield, Wisconsin, the department offers children of all ages individualized weight management help from a multidisciplinary team of medical professionals, including a physician, nurse practitioner, registered dietitian, and sports medicine experts.

Phone: (800) 335-5251 ext. 7-5039

Web site: www.marshfieldclinic.org

New York Comprehensive Weight Control Program

Affiliated with New York–Presbyterian Hospital in New York City, the program offers individual weight management counseling for children, teens, and young adults. It is led by pediatric endocrinologist Ileana Vargas, M.D., and registered dietitian Kathy Isoldi, M.S., C.D.E., who specializes in pediatric care. Their approach involves "dietary adjustment," physical activity, and behavioral guidance. The focus is on individualizing each person's plan, with an emphasis on family involvement.

> **Phone:** (212) 583-1000
> **Web site:** www.weightscience.com

Nutrition Rx

Nutrition Rx is the private practice of nutritionist Alexis Beck, M.P.H., R.D., in Brookline, Massachusetts. She specializes in weight management and diet-related disease prevention. Her approach is to work one-on-one with clients, who typically come to her for weekly one-hour visits. Her motto is "Helping you toward a healthy relationship with food." On an as needed basis, Ms. Beck works with consulting psychiatrists, psychologists, physicians, and fitness experts.

> **Phone:** (617) 731-6786
> **Web site:** www.nutritionrx.com

Prescript Fit Medical Nutrition Therapy System

A program developed by Stanford Owen, M.D., of Gulfport, Mississippi, for people of all ages, this system focuses on health and weight management, using food groups to teach participants about calorie balance and nutrition. The system is self-instructive, with a companion cookbook for each food group, but "coaches" (counselors) are available to ensure compliance with the program. According to Dr. Owen, the system uses nutrition supplements and meal replacement products to improve glucose metabolism, ensure compliance, and lower calorie intake.

Phone: (888) 460-6286

Web site: www.drdiet.com

Saving Our Children

Saving Our Children is a pediatric weight management program developed by Barry Shapiro, M.D., an ear, nose, and throat specialist with a special interest in childhood obesity. It is located in Briarcliff Manor, a northern suburb of New York City. Dr. Shapiro works with young people and their parents, employing a one-on-one approach that makes use of SHAPEDOWN program materials. Dr. Shapiro's program offers strategies to change habits, some supplemental nutrition products, and all-around healthy eating guidelines. It includes recommendations to limit carbohydrates and increase physical activity. Dr. Shapiro emphasizes how important it is for parents to be role models for healthy behavior.

Phone: (914) 944-0531

Web site: www.healthylife2000.net

Virginia Commonwealth University (VCU) Obesity Surgery Center

The center, in Richmond, Virginia, has been performing obesity surgery for more than twenty-five years and is an American Society for Bariatric Surgery Center of Excellence. The multidisciplinary team includes surgeons, registered dietitians, psychologists, registered nurses, and nurse practitioners. The team views surgery as a tool, not a magic cure, for treating obesity. Many teens have been treated here, although the center doesn't cater specifically to teens. A separate adolescent weight management program is offered prior to surgery.

Phone: (804) 828-8000

Web site: www.helpforobesity.com

OTHER WORTHWHILE PROGRAMS

The following programs offer sound approaches but were not used by the teens in this book.

Center for Healthy Weight

The Center for Healthy Weight, at Lucile Packard Children's Hospital at Stanford in Palo Alto, California, was developed and runs under the direction of Thomas Robinson, M.D., and colleagues. It brings together the Stanford University research, patient care and advocacy, public policy, and community programs focused on preventing and treating obesity in children and adolescents. The patient care programs use an interdisciplinary approach based on state-of-the-art research on weight management in young people. They offer a pediatric outpatient weight clinic that provides medical evaluation and individual weight management counseling; a family-based group behavioral weight control program; and an obesity surgery program for teens. A training program for other professionals who wish to start similar programs in their own settings is in development.

Phone: Pediatric weight clinic and bariatric surgery referrals: (650) 736-2114; family-based group behavioral program: (650) 725-4424

Web site: www.healthyweight.lpch.org

Dean Foods LEAN (Lifestyle, Exercise, And Nutrition) Families Program

Sponsored by Children's Medical Center Dallas (in Texas), the program is designed to provide children, teens, and their families with intensive weight management therapy "to support them in achieving and maintaining lifelong habits of good nutrition and healthy activities." The program is run by a multidisciplinary team that involves families in behavioral therapy, physical activity, and nutrition education in twelve weekly group sessions, plus four follow-up sessions. Classes are based on the age, level of understanding, and spoken language of the young person.

Phone: (214) 456-LEAN

Web site: www.childrens.com

Healthy Living Academies

Healthy Living Academies offers several different types of programs for overweight adolescents. All of the programs are designed to provide rapid weight loss through diet and activity management, intensive behavior modification training, parent education, recreational therapy, and an aftercare program. Most of the work with young people is done by master's- and doctoral-level therapists. They help young people who "simply need to learn how to enjoy activity and healthful food," but they also work with those who have emotional and psychological issues that may have contributed to their weight gain. One of the programs is the Academy of the Sierras in Reedley, California. The first boarding school specifically designed to help overweight teens lose weight, it operates year-round and offers a full college preparatory academic program in addition to its multidisciplinary weight loss approach. Healthy Living Academies also operates the Wellspring Camps, described as "the first clinically based summer treatment programs for overweight adolescents and young adults." The camps are located in New York State, North Carolina, California, Michigan, and northern England. (The camp in Michigan is a family camp for kids ages five to thirteen and their parents.)

Phone: (866) 364-0808

Web site: www.healthylivingacademies.com

Pediatric Weight Management Program at the University of Minnesota Children's Hospital

The program offers interdisciplinary care to children and teens who are overweight or obese. Following a medical evaluation by a physician, treatment is tailored to meet individual needs. Options include individual weight management counseling, management of weight-related medical conditions, a group behavioral program, family treatment, and adolescent bariatric surgery. Because this program is part of the University of Minnesota Department of Pediatrics, some patients have the option of participating in ongoing clinical research studies. The Pediatric Weight Management Program also trains professionals to work with children who are overweight.

Phone: (612) 884-0936

Web site: www.uofmchildrenshospital.org/Services/Services/c_1960 74.asp

Internet Resources
for Teens and Parents

With so much health information on the Internet, it's hard to know what's reliable and what's not. I recommend these Web sites for parents, teens, and tweens (kids between the ages of nine and thirteen) who are interested in health, weight management, nutrition, and physical activity. (Some have content in Spanish as well as English.)

This list is by no means exhaustive. I cannot vouch for the validity of all information on these Web sites or those to which they are linked. Because Web sites commonly go out of business, merge with other sites, or move without leaving a forwarding address, some of the Web addresses may no longer be accessible or the content of the sites may have changed. The content here reflects information gathered early in 2006.

www.kidnetic.com

This interactive, noncommercial Web site promotes healthy eating and active living for children ages nine to twelve and their families. A program of the International Food Information Council Foundation, it is funded by the food, beverage, and agricultural industries and was developed in partnership with a number of respected professional organizations. The site offers lots of activities and useful information for both kids and parents, along with a Kidnector, designed to help parents and children talk to one another.

www.teenshealth.org

This Web site was created for teens looking for accurate, honest information and advice about health, relationships, and growing up. Sponsored by the Nemours Foundation, an organization that supports a number of children's health facilities throughout the United States, the site is part of a larger Web site, www.kidshealth.org, with sections for parents and younger kids, too. Content is reviewed by medical professionals.

www.kidsnutrition.org

This site is from the Children's Nutrition Research Center, which is part of a cooperative venture by Baylor College of Medicine, Texas Children's Hospital, and the U.S. Department of Agriculture. Along with articles on various topics and links to other resources, the site has an interactive "healthy eating calculator" that provides a customized general eating plan to help normal-weight children and teens between the ages of four and eighteen eat healthfully without gaining excessive weight. The site also offers a free nutrition newsletter.

www.eatright.org

This is the American Dietetic Association's Web site. Although much of its information is for members only, the site has a consumer resources section that's timely and accurate, as well as a link that helps consumers locate registered dietitians in their area.

www.diabetes.org

The Web site for the American Diabetes Association, it includes a separate area for teens (in the "for parents & kids" link). The site also provides recipes, as well as information about nutrition, weight loss, and exercise.

www.girlshealth.gov (also www.4girls.gov)

Sponsored by the National Women's Health Information Center of the U.S. Department of Health and Human Services, the site was designed for girls between the ages of ten and sixteen and provides reliable information on health topics, including fitness, nutrition, and relationship issues, that concern girls. By using supportive, positive, nonthreatening messages, it tries to motivate girls to choose healthy behaviors.

www.shapingamericasyouth.org

This site has a large registry of programs directed at increasing physical activity and improving nutrition in youth, including some programs for overweight kids. Partners include some respected professional organizations, such as the American Academy of Pediatrics.

www.exhibits.pacsci.org/nutrition

This is an interactive site sponsored by the Pacific Science Center and the Washington State Dairy Council, with games for learning about various aspects of nutrition, weight control, sports nutrition, and more. It allows you to enter gender and age, then put meals together to see how they stack up nutritionally.

www.bam.gov (Body and Mind)

Created by the Centers for Disease Control and Prevention to give kids ages nine to thirteen information for making healthy lifestyle choices, this site focuses on topics such as food and nutrition, safety, stress, and physical activity, using kid-friendly language, games, quizzes, and other interactive features. It has tools to help kids set up their own physical activity routines, as well as a "teacher's corner."

www.girlpower.gov

The Web site for a national campaign sponsored by the U.S. Department of Health and Human Services, it helps encourage nine- to thirteen-year-old girls "to make the most of their lives." With separate areas for grownups and kids, the site offers information on body image, nutrition, fitness, and healthy lifestyle.

www.cookinglight.com
This is the Web site for *Cooking Light* magazine. It provides many healthy recipes as well as nutrition and fitness tips. Some of the content is free and some is not.

www.smallstep.gov
Designed by the U.S. Department of Health and Human Services to help people make gradual, positive changes in their eating and activity habits, the information on this Web site is divided into two main sections: one for adults and teens, the other for younger kids. Resources include an activity tracker, recipes, and a newsletter.

www.verbnow.com
Another interactive Web site by the Centers for Disease Control and Prevention, it was designed for kids between ages nine and thirteen and created "to help children discover the excitement of being active and living a healthy lifestyle." The colorful, entertaining site allows young people to explore new activities and chat with one another about their favorite activities.

www.melpomene.org/girlwise/girlwise.htm
This site is operated by the Melpomene Institute, an organization that provides research on and resources for physical activity and health for girls and women. It addresses topics including physical activity, self-esteem, body image, and nutrition.

www.presidentschallenge.org
The President's Challenge is a program that encourages people of all ages "to make being active part of their everyday lives." The site has a link just for teens and an activity log for tracking progress.

www.tvallowance.com
On this Web site you can purchase a device that allows you to control the amount of time your kids spend watching TV, playing video games, and surfing the Net.

www.tv-turnoff.org
This is the Web site of the TV-Turnoff Network, a nonprofit organization that "encourages children and adults to watch much less television in order to promote healthier lives and communities." It offers practical tips for watching less TV.

http://apps.nccd.cdc.gov/shi
Created as a self-assessment and planning tool, this site was developed by the Centers for Disease Control and Prevention for schools to improve their health and safety policies and programs. It's also useful for parents who want to improve school food and physical activity programs.

www.clinicaltrials.gov
This is a U.S. National Institutes of Health Web site that provides information about federally and privately funded clinical research involving volunteers. If you enter "child obesity" in the search bar, you can find a list of studies that are recruiting young people.

www.readysetgo.org
Sponsored by Canada's Ontario Physical and Health Education Association, this interactive Web site is designed to help children have a healthy sports attitude, as well as recognize the benefits and fun associated with being physically active.

www.activehealthykids.ca
This is the Web site for Active Healthy Kids Canada, a charitable organi-

zation committed to increasing physical activity in children and youth. The group "provides expertise and direction to decision makers at all levels, from policy makers to parents."

www.newmoon.org

New Moon Publishing, which publishes *New Moon* magazine, produces this Web site. The ad-free *New Moon* magazine is edited by and for eight- to fourteen-year-old girls (with the help of an adult staff) and is designed for a multicultural audience. It focuses on contemporary issues that interest girls and emphasize nonappearance-related accomplishments.

www.actionforhealthykids.com

Operated by a public-private nonprofit partnership of many U.S. organizations and government agencies, this site is designed to address weight problems and undernourishment by focusing on changes in schools. It provides resources to improve schools and links so users can find out what's going on in schools in their state.

Web Sites Recommended by the Teens

Following is a list of Web sites that the teens found helpful for weight management. A number of them are not geared specifically to teens, but they may have some useful information for young people. Inclusion in this list does not necessarily indicate my own endorsement, nor does it necessarily indicate that all the advice on the sites is reliable. Teen readers and their parents need to assess whether these resources suit their circumstances. Note, too, that some of the Web sites in this section have pop-up ads or links that are inappropriate or promote certain products that I do not recommend. This information was gathered early in 2006; some of these sites and their content will change with time.

When going to any health-related Web site, it's important to try to find out if the content is reliable. See if the site is run and reviewed by health professionals, such as experts in the field, medical centers, the government, or other respected organizations. Always be careful about giving out any personal information and check out a site's privacy policy. If a site offers chat rooms or any sort of online community, check to see who's involved and who's moderating things. Beware that chat sessions with lay members of an online community may not offer legitimate advice. Finally, take into consideration the sources of funding for the site and, for sites at which you pay for services, read the terms of the contract carefully before committing.

www.ivillage.com

This large online community primarily targets adult women, although it does provide some content aimed at teens and parents of teens. Health and nutrition topics are covered.

www.nutritiondata.com

This site provides nutrition facts for foods and recipes and also allows users to track total calorie consumption.

www.prevention.com

The Web site for *Prevention* magazine, it is primarily geared to adult women. Entering "teens" into the site's search engine brings up links to many articles on parenting of teens.

www.toneteen.com

This site was developed by a previously overweight teen who is now a certified personal fitness trainer. She shares her story and provides free access to nutrition and fitness information that comes from various sources.

www.dwlz.com

"Dotti's Weight Loss Zone" reflects the experiences of its developer, a woman who has lost weight. She gives updates on her progress, sells downloadable books with recipes in them, holds online seminars, and offers restaurant and food nutrition information, as well as much more.

www.skinnydailypost.com

A group blog started by several people who have lost weight, this site provides "short, daily essays on weight loss and fitness from people who have been there, done that, and work hard every day to keep their weight off."

www.ediets.com

This Web site offers many personalized online weight loss and nutrition programs, including an online version of the Trim Kids program (see page 210), as well as support boards for parents. Some of the nutrition information at eDiets is free, but there is a fee for the weight loss programs.

Selected References

"Adolescent Nutrition: A Springboard for Health." *Journal of the American Dietetic Association* 102, no. 3, Suppl. (2002).

American Academy of Pediatrics. "Identifying and Treating Eating Disorders." *Pediatrics* 111, no. 1 (2003): 204–11.

American Academy of Pediatrics. "Preventing Childhood Obesity: A National Conference Focusing on Pregnancy, Infancy, and Early Childhood Factors." *Pediatrics* 114, no. 4, Suppl. (2004).

American Academy of Pediatrics. "Treatment of Overweight Children and Adolescents: A Needs Assessment of Health Practitioners." *Pediatrics* 110, no. 1, Suppl. (2002).

American Dietetic Association. "Childhood Overweight." Evidence Analysis Library, 2004. http://www.eatright.org.

————. "Position of the American Dietetic Association: Individual-, Family-, School-, and Community-Based Interventions for Pediatric Overweight." *Journal of the American Dietetic Association* 106, no. 6 (2006): 925–45.

Astrup, Arne, Thomas M. Larsen, and Angela Harper. "Atkins and Other Low-Carbohydrate Diets: Hoax or an Effective Tool for Weight Loss?" *Lancet* 364 (2004): 897–99.

Barlow, Sarah E., and William H. Dietz. "Obesity Evaluation and Treatment: Expert Committee Recommendations." *Pediatrics* 102, no. 3 (1998): 1–11.

Barr, Susan I. "Increased Dairy Product or Calcium Intake: Is Body Weight or Composition Affected in Humans?" *Journal of Nutrition* 133, no. 1 (2003): 245S–48S.

Berg-Smith, S. M., V. J. Stevens, K. M. Brown, L. Van Horn, N. Gernhofer, E. Peters, R. Greenberg, L. Snetselaar, L. Ahrens, and K. Smith. "A Brief Motivational Intervention to Improve Dietary Adherence in Adolescents." *Health Education Research* 14, no. 3 (1999): 399–410.

Berkowitz, Robert I., Thomas A. Wadden, Andrew M. Tershakovec, and Joanna L. Cronquist. "Behavior Therapy and Sibutramine for the Treatment of Adolescent Obesity." *Journal of the American Medical Association* 289, no. 14 (2003): 1805–12.

Birch, Leann L., and Jennifer O. Fisher. "Development of Eating Behaviors Among Children and Adolescents." *Pediatrics* 101, no. 3 (1998): 539–49.

Birch, Leann L., Jennifer O. Fisher, and Kirsten K. Davison. "Learning to Overeat: Maternal Use of Restrictive Feeding Practices Promotes Girls' Eating in the Absence of Hunger." *American Journal of Clinical Nutrition* 78, no. 2 (2003): 215–20.

Braet, Caroline. "Patient Characteristics as Predictors of Weight Loss After an Obesity Treatment for Children." *Obesity* 14, no. 1 (2006): 148–55.

Brown, Judith E., Janet S. Isaacs, U. Beate Krinke, Maureen A. Murtaugh, Jamie Stang, and Nancy H. Wooldridge. *Nutrition Through the Life Cycle.* Belmont, Calif.: Wadsworth Thomson Learning, 2004.

Butryn, Meghan L., and Thomas A. Wadden. "Treatment of Overweight in Children and Adolescents: Does Dieting Increase the Risk of Eating Disorders?" *International Journal of Eating Disorders* 37, no. 4 (2005): 285–93.

Canadian Association of Paediatric Health Centres, Paediatric Chairs of Canada, and Canadian Institutes of Health Research. *Addressing Childhood Obesity: The Evidence for Action,* 2004.

Dalton, Sharron. *Our Overweight Children.* Berkeley: University of California Press, 2004.

Daniels, Stephen R., Donna K. Arnett, Robert H. Eckel, Samuel S. Gidding, Laura L. Hayman, Shiriki Kumanyika, Thomas N. Robinson, Barbara J. Scott, Sachiko St. Jeor, and Christine L. Williams. "Overweight in Children and Adolescents: Pathophysiology, Consequences, Prevention, and Treatment." *Circulation* 111 no. 15 (2005): 1999–2012.

Developing Adolescents: A Reference for Professionals. Washington, D.C.: American Psychological Association, 2002.

Ebbeling, Cara B., Michael M. Leidig, Kelly B. Sinclair, Jan P. Hangen, and David S. Ludwig. "A Reduced-Glycemic Load Diet in the Treatment of Adolescent Obesity." *Archives of Pediatrics and Adolescent Medicine* 157, no. 8 (2003): 773–79.

Ebbeling, Cara B., Kelly B. Sinclair, Mark A. Pereira, Erica Garcia-Lago, Henry A. Feldman, and David S. Ludwig. "Compensation for Energy Intake from Fast Food Among Overweight and Lean Adolescents." *Journal of the American Medical Association* 291, no. 23 (2004): 2828–33.

Eisenberg, Marla E., Dianne Neumark-Sztainer, and Mary Story. "Associations of Weight-Based Teasing and Emotional Well-Being Among Adolescents." *Archives of Pediatrics and Adolescent Medicine* 157, no. 8 (2003): 733–38.

Epstein, Leonard H., and Gary S. Goldfield. "Physical Activity in the Treatment of Childhood Overweight and Obesity: Current Evidence and Research Issues." *Medicine and Science in Sports and Exercise* 31, no. 11 (1999): S553–59.

Epstein, Leonard H., Constance C. Gordy, Hollie A. Raynor, Marlene Beddome, Colleen K. Kilanowski, and Rocco Paluch. "Increasing Fruit and Vegetable Intake and Decreasing Fat and Sugar Intake in Families at Risk for Childhood Obesity." *Obesity Research* 9, no. 3 (2001): 171–78.

Epstein, Leonard H., Michelle D. Myers, Hollie A. Raynor, and Brian E. Saelens. "Treatment of Pediatric Obesity." *Pediatrics* 101, no. 3 Suppl. (1998): 554–70.

Epstein, Leonard H., James N. Roemmich, and Hollie A. Raynor. "Behavioral Therapy in the Treatment of Pediatric Obesity." *Pediatric Clinics of North America* 48, no. 4 (2001): 981–93.

Epstein, Leonard H., Alice Valoski, Rena R. Wing, and James McCurley. "Ten-Year Outcomes of Behavioral Family-Based Treatment for Childhood Obesity." *Health Psychology* 13, no. 5 (1994): 373–83.

Field, Alison, S. B. Austin, C. B. Taylor, Susan Malspeis, Bernard Rosner, Helaine R. Rockett, Matthew W. Gillman, and Graham A. Colditz. "Relation Between Dieting and Weight Change Among Preadolescents and Adolescents." *Pediatrics* 112, no. 4 (2003): 900–6.

Fisher, J. O., and L. L. Birch. "Restricting Access to Foods and Children's Eating." *Appetite* 32, no. 3 (1999): 405–19.

Gordon-Larsen, Penny, Linda S. Adair, Melissa C. Nelson, and Barry M. Popkin. "Five-Year Obesity Incidence in the Transition Period Between Adolescence and Adulthood: The National Longitudinal Study of Adolescent Health." *American Journal of Clinical Nutrition* 80, no. 1 (2004): 1–7.

Grobman, K. H. "Diana Baumrind's Theory of Parenting Styles: Original Descriptions of the Styles." http://devpsy.org/teaching/parent/baumrind_styles.html.

Harrell, Joanne S., Robert G. McMurray, Christopher D. Baggett, Michael L. Pennell, Patricia F. Pearce, and Shrikant I. Bangdiwala. "Energy Costs of Physical Activities in Children and Adolescents." *Medicine and Science in Sports and Exercise* 37, no. 2 (2005): 329–36.

Hsu, George L. K. "Epidemiology of the Eating Disorders." *Psychiatric Clinics of North America* 19, no. 4 (1996): 681–700.

Ikeda, Joanne. *If My Child Is Overweight, What Should I Do About It?* Rev. ed. Oakland: University of California Agriculture and Natural Resources, 2004.

Inge, Thomas H., Nancy F. Krebs, Victor F. Garcia, Joseph A. Skelton, Karen S. Guice, Richard S. Strauss, Craig T. Albanese, Mary L.

Brandt, Lawrence D. Hammer, Carol M. Harmon, Timothy D. Kane, William J. Klish, Keith T. Oldham, Colin D. Rudolph, Michael A. Helmrath, Edward Donovan, and Stephen R. Daniels. "Bariatric Surgery for Severely Overweight Adolescents: Concerns and Recommendations." *Pediatrics* 114, no. 1 (2004): 217–23.

Institute of Medicine of the National Academies. *Dietary Reference Intakes for Energy, Carbohydrate, Fiber, Fat, Fatty Acids, Cholesterol, Protein, and Amino Acids: Part 1.* Washington, D.C.: National Academies Press, 2002.

Institute of Medicine of the National Academies. *Preventing Childhood Obesity.* Washington, D.C.: National Academies Press, 2005.

Jelalian, Elissa, and Brian E. Saelens. "Empirically Supported Treatments in Pediatric Psychology: Pediatric Obesity." *Journal of Pediatric Psychology* 24, no. 3 (1999): 223–48.

Johnson, Susan L. "Improving Preschoolers' Self-Regulation of Energy Intake." *Pediatrics* 106, no. 6 (2000): 1429–35.

Kaiser Family Foundation. "Generation M: Media in the Lives of 8–18-Year-Olds," 2005. http://www.kff.org/entmedia/entmedia030905nr.cfm.

Kimm, Sue Y. S., Nancy W. Glynn, Eva Obarzanek, Andrea M. Kriska, Stephen R. Daniels, Bruce A. Barton, and Kiang Liu. "Relation Between the Changes in Physical Activity and Body-Mass Index During Adolescence: A Multicentre Longitudinal Study." *Lancet* 366, no. 9482 (2005): 301–7.

Kirk, Shelley, Barbara J. Scott, and Stephen R. Daniels. "Pediatric Obesity Epidemic: Treatment Options." *Journal of the American Dietetic Association* 105, no. 5 (2005): S44–51.

Kirschenbaum, Daniel S., Julie N. Germann, and Barry H. Rich. "Treatment of Morbid Obesity in Low-Income Adolescents: Effects of Parental Self-Monitoring." *Obesity Research* 13, no. 9 (2005): 1527–29.

Makino, Mariko, Koji Tsuboi, and Lorraine Dennerstein. "Prevalence of

Eating Disorders: A Comparison of Western and Non-Western Countries." *Medscape General Medicine* 6, no. 3. (2004). http://medscape.com/viewarticle/487413.

Maziekas, M. T., L. M. LeMura, N. M. Stoddard, S. Kaercher, and T. Martucci. "Follow Up Exercise Studies in Paediatric Obesity: Implications for Long Term Effectiveness." *British Journal of Sports Medicine* 37, no. 5 (2003): 425–29.

Mullen, Mary C., and Jodie Shield. *Childhood and Adolescent Overweight.* Chicago: American Dietetic Association, 2004.

Neumark-Sztainer, Dianne. "Dieting and Binge Eating Among Adolescents: What Do They Really Mean?" *Journal of the American Dietetic Association* 98, no. 4 (1998): 446–50.

———. *"I'm, Like, SO Fat!" Helping Your Teen Make Healthy Choices About Eating and Exercise in a Weight-Obsessed World.* New York: Guilford Press, 2005.

———. "Obesity and Eating Disorder Prevention: An Integrated Approach?" *Adolescent Medicine: State of the Art Reviews* 14, no. 1 (2003): 159–73.

———. "Recommendations from Overweight Youth Regarding School-Based Weight Control Programs." *Journal of School Health* 67, no. 10 (1997): 428–33.

Neumark-Sztainer, Dianne, Peter J. Hannan, Mary Story, and Cheryl L. Perry. "Weight-Control Behaviors Among Adolescent Girls and Boys: Implications for Dietary Intake." *Journal of the American Dietetic Association* 104, no. 6 (2004): 913–20.

Neumark-Sztainer, Dianne, Mary Story, Peter J. Hannan, Cheryl L. Perry, and Lori M. Irving. "Weight-Related Concerns and Behaviors Among Overweight and Nonoverweight Adolescents." *Archives of Pediatrics and Adolescent Medicine* 156, no. 2 (2002): 171–78.

Neumark-Sztainer, Dianne, Mary Story, Cheryl Perry, and Mary Anne Casey. "Factors Influencing Food Choices of Adolescents: Findings from Focus-Group Discussions with Adolescents." *Journal of the American Dietetic Association* 99, no. 8 (1999): 929–34.

Neumark-Sztainer, Dianne, Melanie Wall, Jia Guo, Mary Story, Jess Haines, and Maria Eisenberg. "Obesity, Disordered Eating, and Eating Disorders in a Longitudinal Study of Adolescents: How Do Dieters Fare 5 Years Later?" *Journal of the American Dietetic Association* 106, no. 4 (2006): 559–68.

Ogden, Cynthia L., Margaret D. Carroll, Lester R. Curtin, Margaret A. McDowell, Carolyn J. Tabak, and Katherine M. Flegal. "Prevalence of Overweight and Obesity in the United States, 1999–2004." *Journal of the American Medical Association* 295, no. 13 (2006): 1549–55.

"Position of the American Dietetic Association: Nutrition Intervention in the Treatment of Anorexia Nervosa, Bulimia Nervosa, and Eating Disorders Not Otherwise Specified (EDNOS)." *Journal of the American Dietetic Association* 101, no. 7 (2001): 810–19.

"Position of the American Dietetic Association: Use of Nutritive and Nonnutritive Sweeteners." *Journal of the American Dietetic Association* 104, no. 2 (2004): 255–68.

Rampersaud, Gail C., Mark A. Pereira, Beverly L. Girard, Judi Adams, and Jordan D. Metzl. "Breakfast Habits, Nutritional Status, Body Weight, and Academic Performance in Children and Adolescents." *Journal of the American Dietetic Association* 105, no. 5 (2005): 743–60.

Robert Wood Johnson Foundation, American Stroke Association, and American Heart Association. *A Nation at Risk: Obesity in the United States,* 2005.

Robinson, Thomas N. "Behavioural Treatment of Childhood and Adolescent Obesity." *International Journal of Obesity* 23, Suppl. 2 (1999): S52–57.

Robinson, Thomas N., Michaela Kiernan, Donna M. Matheson, and K. Farish Haydel. "Is Parental Control over Children's Eating Associated with Childhood Obesity? Results from a Population-Based Sample of Third Graders." *Obesity Research* 9, no. 5 (2001): 306–12.

Rolls, Barbara J. "The Supersizing of America." *Nutrition Today* 38, no. 2 (2003): 42–53.

Rolls, Barbara J., Adam Drewnowski, and Jenny H. Ledikwe. "Changing the Energy Density of the Diet as a Strategy for Weight Management." *Journal of the American Dietetic Association* 105, no. 5 (2005): S98–103.

Saelens, Brian E., and Ann M. McGrath. "Self-Monitoring Adherence and Adolescent Weight Control Efficacy." *Children's Health Care* 32, no. 2 (2003): 137–52.

Satter, Ellyn M. "Internal Regulation and the Evolution of Normal Growth as the Basis for Prevention of Obesity in Children." *Journal of the American Dietetic Association* 96, no. 9 (1996): 860–64.

Shunk, Jennifer A., and Leann L. Birch. "Girls at Risk for Overweight at Age 5 Are at Risk for Dietary Restraint, Disinhibited Overeating, Weight Concerns, and Greater Weight Gain from 5 to 9 Years." *Journal of the American Dietetic Association* 104, no. 7 (2004): 1120–26.

Slavin, Joanne L. "Dietary Fiber and Body Weight." *Nutrition* 21, no. 3 (2005): 411–18.

Sothern, Melinda S., T. Kristian von Almen, and Heidi Schumacher. *Trim Kids.* New York: Quill, 2001.

Stang, Jamie, Johanna Rehorst, and Maggie Golicic. "Parental Feeding Practices and Risk of Childhood Overweight in Girls: Implications for Dietetics Practice." *Journal of the American Dietetic Association* 104, no. 7 (2004): 1076–79.

Stice, Eric, Rebecca P. Cameron, Chris Hayward, C. Barr Taylor, and Joel D. Killen. "Naturalistic Weight-Reduction Efforts Prospectively Predict Growth in Relative Weight and Onset of Obesity

Among Female Adolescents." *Journal of Consulting and Clinical Psychology* 67, no. 6 (1999): 967–74.

Story, Mary, Dianne Neumark-Sztainer, Nancy Sherwood, Jamie Stang, and David Murray. "Dieting Status and Its Relationship to Eating and Physical Activity Behaviors in a Representative Sample of US Adolescents." *Journal of the American Dietetic Association* 99, no. 4 (1999): 1127–36.

Strong, William B., Robert M. Malina, Cameron R. Blimkie, Stephen R. Daniels, Rodney K. Dishman, Bernard Gutin, Albert C. Hergenroeder, Aviva Must, Patricia A. Nixon, James M. Pivarnik, Thomas Rowland, Steward Trost, and François Trudeau. "Evidence Based Physical Activity for School-Age Youth." *Journal of Pediatrics* (2005): 732–37.

Summerbell, C. D., V. Ashton, K. J. Campbell, L. Edmunds, S. Kelly, and E. Waters. "Interventions for Treating Obesity in Children." Cochrane Database of Systematic Reviews, 2004.

Thompson, Kevin J., and Linda Smolak, eds. *Body Image, Eating Disorders, and Obesity in Youth.* Washington, D.C.: American Psychological Association, 2001.

U.S. Department of Health and Human Services and Centers for Disease Control and Prevention. "Youth Risk Behavior Surveillance — United States, 2003." *Morbidity and Mortality Weekly Report* 53, no. SS-2 (2004).

U.S. Department of Health and Human Services and U.S. Department of Agriculture. *Dietary Guidelines for Americans,* 2005.

Wadden, Thomas A., and Albert J. Stunkard, eds. *Handbook of Obesity Treatment.* New York: Guilford Press, 2002.

Zametkin, Alan J., Christine K. Zoon, Hannah W. Klein, and Suzanne Munson. "Psychiatric Aspects of Child and Adolescent Obesity: A Review of the Past 10 Years." *Journal of the American Academy of Child and Adolescent Psychiatry* 43, no. 2 (2004): 134–53.

Index